Triumph Over Cancer

A Natural Approach

by Agi Lidle

A Better Life Publications
❖ Scottsdale

Contents

Lidle Café Cookbook   page 127

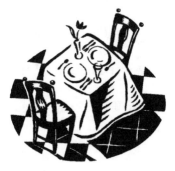

Thank You Everyone

*f*or the encouragement and inspiration you've given me through my incredible healing journey. Recently I heard the statement, "Adversity introduces us to ourselves." This is certainly true, because cancer introduced me to a side of myself I never knew existed. A determined and courageous side that isn't afraid of cancer. The winning side that is armed with the knowledge to defeat it.

This book is dedicated to all people seeking
to live a long and healthy life.

Planting Seeds of Change

Triumph Over Cancer is not just another book about health. It is written by Agi Lidle, a cancer survivor and certified herbalist, who has become an expert in her own healing experience.

She has experienced one extreme of living to the other extreme... from obsessively over eating... to living a balanced and healthy lifestyle.

Agi shares the intimate details of her life and the factors leading up to the diagnosis of cancer. Factors including: a dysfunctional childhood, unreleased emotions of unforgiveness, enormous stress, and her unhealthy diet.

The book reveals the tools necessary for achieving and maintaining a healthy lifestyle. Agi began her healing journey by making simple changes in her life. By following the basic Natural Health Principles outlined in this book, she cleansed her body from years of accumulated mucus and toxins. With great determination, she built her immune system to a level where cancer couldn't exist any longer.

A great benefit to the reader is her detailed shopping list, it takes the guessing out of shopping for healthy foods. By popular demand, her favorite recipes are also featured.

This powerful and encouraging book will enable the reader to live a healthier future by making more informed choices.

Adversity
Introduces Us
To
Ourselves

For whatever reason you have chosen to read this book, my hope is that it be of great benefit and inspiration to you.

Everything I'm sharing in this book is true. It all happened to me. If someone were to tell me four and a half years ago that I would have breast cancer, be healed from breast cancer naturally, change my fast food lifestyle, and be spiritually renewed...I wouldn't have believed it.

In the same way, the terrorist attack on the Twin Towers and the Pentagon made us realize how vulnerable we are as a society.....we are just as vulnerable to cancer's terrorist attack on our bodies and minds. Cancer lays dormant (like the terrorist sleeper cells) until our defense is down and then it strikes.

How and when we choose to deal with cancer is vital to our well-being. Unfortunately, many of us let our defenses down. We must gain the knowledge to build our immune systems, which are our first line of defense. With a strong immune system, if cancer were to invade our body...it can eliminate and guard it from future attacks.

The human body has been designed to fight disease and heal itself, if it is prepared. I've experienced the magnificence of my immune system in action. With proper nourishment and support, it was able to fight cancer and win.

If I can make the changes in my lifestyle to be healthy, energetic and mentally clear...you can too. It's worth the effort.

Chapter One

Life Before Cancer

Dysfunctional, with a capital 'D' just about sums it up.

Much of my childhood is a blurred memory. It wasn't a happy one, so I've suppressed most of it. Writing this book is a wonderful form of therapy. I'm surprised I'm sharing so many personal details of my life.

Before I share my healing experience and exactly how I achieved it, it's important for you to understand my life before cancer.

I'll begin by telling you about my mother and father, Klara and Joseph Barsi. They met on a train, fleeing Communist Hungary during the revolution in 1956. Both were only nineteen years old and eager to experience their newfound freedom. They would first settle in France and as soon as they could get visas, they would go to the United States.

Within a few months of their arrival in France they were married. Almost immediately afterwards, my father began to drink heavily and would disappear for days at a time. When he finally came home my mother always confronted him. Her confrontations always led to shouting and screaming, inevitably ending in physical and emotional abuse. *My mother was pregnant with my brother, Barna during these violent episodes.*

Barna was born on September 17, 1957 and I was born on September 4, 1958. In those days abuse wasn't talked about. It was hidden away like dirty laundry.

I can remember my mother being outgoing, full of life, and filled with endless energy. Everyone liked her and she had many friends. Playful at heart and free spirited, she never failed to take my brother and I on an adventure almost every weekend. My mother was like a breath of fresh air. She loved life. Whatever she set her mind out to do, she did.

On the other hand, my father was an introvert with few close friends and never attempted to make new ones. He rarely had anything nice to say about anyone and thought all were out to cheat him. My father had absolutely no respect for women and as far as he was concerned, all women to him were "whores."

My father was born and raised in Communist Hungary, without knowing his father. School kids made fun of him for being fatherless and even some of his teachers treated him unfairly. At a very early age he had to defend himself against this discrimination. Unfortunately, the only way he knew how to deal with this was through violence.

I believe he grew up feeling deep resentment for his mother, blaming her for his fathers' abandonment.

Somehow, my mother's spirit managed to survive all of the abuse and her dream to live in America was about to come true. In 1964 it was difficult to get a visa to the United States, but that didn't stop my mother. At last, after months of endless effort she was granted our visas.

My brother was six and I was five when we arrived in New York City. My mother really did believe that if she could make it in New York City she could make it anywhere. She hoped this was a new beginning for our family and the abuse would stop. Sadly, it didn't. The abuse continued and became even more unbearable.

My father was not only abusing her, but now he was beginning to emotionally abuse my brother.

We never knew if or when my father was coming home, and whether he would be drunk. The days when he did come home almost always ended in physical or verbal abuse. My brother and I would literally shake with fear anticipating the inevitable abuse against our mother.

Throughout my childhood years, I suffered with continuous stomach problems that I now know were caused from fear for my mother and brother's safety. Each time my mother and father began to fight I began to cry, hoping all attention would shift to me and the fighting would stop. It seemed to work for a while, but as the years went by nothing helped stop the abuse.

Amazingly enough, my father never physically abused me. Probably because I was always sick and he must have felt sorry for me. I was his 'little girl' and in his own dysfunctional way he loved me, and I knew it. The abuse I endured growing up was watching my mother and brother suffer. Witnessing their spirits slowly die.

At five years old, I developed a nervous twitch and uncontrollable head shaking. My parents thought it was another ploy for me to get them to stop fighting, *but it wasn't.*

After many months, my mother realized something was really wrong with me and took me to see a doctor. The doctor didn't know what it was and told her I would out grow it. *I didn't out grow it* and my mother loathed my father even more because she blamed him for my condition.

My brother was eleven and I was ten, when my mother moved us cross-country to Arizona, to begin a new life without my father. A few months later, he followed us and wormed his way back into our lives with temporary kindness and empty promises of reform.

We wanted to believe him. After all he was our father. For a few months he really did change. Until one night when our friends, who were also Hungarian, were over for dinner and my father began to drink. He violently assaulted my mother by throwing a cast iron skillet at her head. She was about eight feet away from him and somehow moved just in time to escape the blow. She ran from him screaming, "Call the police, call the police."

The police arrived and talked to him outside and tried to calm him down. He wasn't arrested, but instead was urged to leave us alone and stay away for a few days.

That was just enough time for my mother to pack his belongings and throw them out the front door. After two days, he came back and my mother wouldn't let him inside our house. All three of us were shaking with fear as we listened to him shouting obscenities outside. The last thing we heard my father say was that he was going to kill my mother by pouring acid on her face.

For months we lived in terror. My mother knew the only way to protect us was to divorce him. When I turned 15 years old the divorce became final. It was at that time in my life I ceased to believe in God. My prayers for my family were not answered, so what was the use?

After the divorce, my father moved to California. The last words I spoke to him were, *"I hate you. You are not my father any more."* I severed all communication with him for almost fourteen years. My brother, on the other hand, stayed in contact.

In May of 1989, Barna called me and said he had just seen our father and he wanted us to visit him. I was shocked, yet extremely excited. He was still my father and even though a part of me hated him, another part of me loved him and always would. I agreed to go because after fourteen years it was time to forgive. A few weeks later, we were on our way to visit my father, my half sister Judith and Marie (my father's new wife). *I had never met either one before.*

During the short four days I spent with my father and sister, an enormous amount of healing occurred, both for my brother and myself. My father told me he was sorry for being such a bad father and even though he didn't show it he always loved me. We embraced and told each other, *"I love you"* countless times.

I knew my father finally gave my brother the love and approval he so desperately wanted. They embraced as well. And what can I say about my little sister...she reminded me of me and I loved her as if I knew her my entire life.

As my brother and I were saying our goodbye, Judith pulled me to the side and whispered in my ear, "Agi, I'm afraid, take me with you." I asked her what she was afraid of and she replied. "I'm afraid father's going to do something bad." I reassured her by telling her, "when I was growing up he used to threaten my family, but he never carried out his threats."

One week after my brother and I left them, my father did the unimaginable. In a fit of insanity, my father shot Marie in the hallway and then proceeded to enter Judith's room as she was sleeping and shot her too, killing them both. Judith was only eleven years old.

He then poured gasoline over their bodies and lit them on fire. Afterwards, my father went into the garage where he committed suicide by shooting himself in the head.

I found out later, the child protective service was on the verge of removing my sister from her home. Their neighbor said they heard my father threaten Marie several times by saying he was going to kill her. My father probably thought, *"If I can't keep my little girl, no one can."*

A Bit More About My Mother

My mother never remarried. I think it's because after the divorce my brother began to drink heavily. She never knew when he would show up unannounced at her home drunk. Often times she would get a phone call from the police station to come get him.

She provided him shelter, when it either got too cold or too hot for him to be on the streets. My mother often told me she couldn't help herself. By continually taking him in, she was enabling him even more to depend on her. "I'm his mother and he has no-one, but me", she would say.

One day my mother just couldn't take it anymore and felt herself on the brink of a nervous breakdown. Thank God for her spirit of survival because she began to read books about the power of the mind. My mother became so fascinated with this subject that she read every book ever written about the mind and didn't have time to have the nervous breakdown.

About My Brother, Barna

My brother and I were really close as children and we looked out for each other's safety (me more than him because by the time Barna was seven he was already getting into trouble. I chose to be the mother hen hovering about him). Barna was a sad little boy who received excruciating emotional whippings from my father. *"You're nothing, you'll never amount to anything"*, he said to my brother. Barna just stood there, trying to hold back the tears from running down his little innocent face. When he couldn't hold them back any longer he ran into his room and cried himself to sleep.

Barna lived for my father's approval and sadly never received it as a child. My mother did the best she could, but there wasn't any substitution for a father's love and approval. So, Barna acted out his hurt and anger by rebelling against everything and everyone. By his senior year of high school he began to drink and within a few years, he became an alcoholic.

Through the years he attended AA programs, detox centers and even spent time in jail, but nothing worked. He couldn't stop drinking. He lived much of his adult life homeless and on the streets. On March 3, 1995, he drowned. He was drunk and fell into a canal.

It's very sad my brother never had self-respect or self-confidence. He was so intelligent and possessed a photographic memory. His heart was as tender and loving as a newborn baby's smile. My brother was a fine person who just didn't know how to live.

I am so grateful that I saw him just days before his death and was able to tell him, *"I love you, Barna."* Today, I'm at peace and free from guilt, knowing I told my brother I loved him before he died. "My brother's spirit lives, and one day I will be re-united with him. *I Love You, Barna."*

About Me

As you already know, I had stomach problems my entire life and at the age of five I began to twitch and shake my head uncontrollably. Have you been able to guess what the twitching and head shaking was a result of?

If you guessed Tourette's syndrome, you're right. When I was ten years old our family doctor made the diagnosis. My mother and I were so relieved because at last we knew what we were dealing with.

Recently, I read an article linking Tourette's to an infection. Researchers think a virus is the cause. Merritt McDinney of the Medical Tribune Times Services writes, "Genetics are believed to play a role in the development of Tourette's syndrome – a condition characterized by involuntary movements as well as bursts of grunts and words." The article continues to read, "Dr. Singer, professor of neurology at Johns Hopkins University School of Medicine, suspects that a bacterial infection may trigger the condition in some genetically susceptible children. One bacterium under suspicion is streptococcus, commonly known as strep."

I've read several theories relating to the cause of Tourette's, but so far no one knows for sure what it is. It feels like the neurotransmitters in my brain are misfiring and firing too often. I've got too much activity in my brain causing mixed signals. The result is involuntary and uncontrollable physical movements, verbal outbursts, obsessive-compulsive behavior and a very short attention span (ADD).

(Later in the book I'll share with you how my healthy diet helps minimize Tourette's symptoms and dramatically reduces ADD, associated with Tourette's syndrome) Some of my past severe symptoms included: constant throat clearing, vocal outbursts (grunts and barks), eye blinking, head shaking and foul language (I tried to keep them under my breath but once in a while one slipped out and always at the wrong time).

I was given the prescription drug Haldal, which turned out to be a horrible drug with horrendous side effects. I stopped taking Haldal after only a few weeks and have not taken any prescription drugs since.

The obsessive-compulsive symptoms (usually associated with Tourette's) were frustrating. When the compulsion manifested itself, I felt like I was stuck in that particular physical act. I couldn't get "unstuck" until the physical act was completed.

Here's an example of one of my obsessive-compulsive episodes... *when I was about ten, my compulsion was to stick out my tongue as far as it would go. The obsession was to keep doing it until I was sure I couldn't stick it out any further. Can you imagine how much trouble this got me into? People thought I was sticking my tongue out at them! It's kind of funny to me now, but it wasn't funny back then. I felt embarrassed and frustrated.*

Another obsessive-compulsive act that lasted for many years was... *before I could open my car door I had to touch the door handle with my wrist. If it didn't touch the door handle just right I got stuck. This was really aggravating because I couldn't get unstuck, until I did it just right. It usually took at least ten efforts before I could open the car door.*

Tourette's syndrome didn't bother me as much during my grade school years. High school was more difficult because I wanted so much to be accepted and popular. I didn't know if I could be accepted having Tourette's. God must have been looking out for me because I was blessed with a wonderful boyfriend and friends throughout my high school years. They saw past these bizarre symptoms and loved me for who I was.

My overall physical health seemed to be fine until I turned sixteen years old. It was during the final tryouts for the cheerleading team *(which I had been assured I made)* when I blew out my knee! Within a week I had surgery to repair the torn cartilage. I was told I wouldn't be able to be physically active for a month or so. My dream of becoming a cheerleader was over.

Later that same year, I developed infectious hepatitis. I was bedridden for an entire month (I contracted it from a girl I worked with who contracted it from her little daughter). I didn't know then that liver damage could result from hepatitis. If I had, I may have been more careful about what I ate and drank in the future.

I felt healthy for the next ten years. The only problems I had; were stomach pains from time to time and allergies during allergy season, which were alleviated with a shot almost every month. Just after my twenty-seventh birthday my health took a turn for the worse.

One morning my kidney area was unusually sensitive. By the end of the day, it felt as if someone was stabbing me with a hot cattle prod. Fortunately, I was dating a physician at the time and he knew immediately it was E.coli. He rushed me to the hospital and gave me the proper medication.

At the age of thirty-two, I had an operation to repair a hernia. The surgery went well and I was up and around the next day.

My Diet…Before Cancer

Hindsight really is 20-20. If I knew then what I know now, I'm certain many of my medical emergencies could have been avoided by simply changing my diet. I've never known anyone who ate as much junk food as I have throughout my life. My mother, bless her heart, tried to feed us nutritional meals whenever she could. Unfortunately, she had to be both the emotional and financial support in our household. By the time she got home from work she was exhausted.

Frozen dinners were extremely popular with my brother and I during the weekdays. On weekends my mother baked delicious homemade Hungarian pastries. Baking comforted her and served as an escape during hard times. Baking also gave my mother, brother and I something to do together, and afforded us a sense of family.

I became a sugar addict at a very early age. Into my twenties Dr. Pepper became my morning addiction as did chocolate. Brushing my teeth before drinking my soda was unthinkable. (Now, it makes me almost nauseous thinking about it). Cappuccino was my discovery and morning addiction into my 30's. I couldn't start my day without the help of the caffeine.

Being a non-cook, my choices were limited to eating out. Mostly fast foods! The few things I ate at home were white bread baguettes, cheeses, grilled steak and potatoes, sausages, pork chops, instant boxed side dishes or micro-waved foods, all desserts and very little salad. Whenever I fixed a salad, it usually had sliced beef on top. Lots of canned soup. (I won't mention the name brand, but all of their soups have MSG on the label). I drank very little water and suffered from constipation most of my adult life (never realizing that going every other day was NOT NORMAL!)

One and a Half Years, Before Cancer

Shortly after my brother Barna's death, I began to have frequent bladder infections. *For years I've been complaining to my gynecologist about the pains in my stomach, but pap smears and physical examinations never revealed any abnormalities. Although, he did urge me to eat more fruits, but I never listened.*

I also started getting dizzy spells and the palms of my hands and the soles of my feet would sweat. I thought I was having anxiety attacks as a result of Barna's death. One day the dizzy spell got so bad that I went to an emergency center. After giving a urine sample the tests revealed sugar in my urine. The doctor was alarmed and wanted me to test for diabetes. I told him I would come back, and never did.

Thinking I probably had diabetes, I began to cut down on my consumption of meat and alcohol. I even started eating healthier foods. The bladder infections went away and the dizzy spells came less often, but something else was beginning to happen. By three o'clock in the afternoon I felt exhausted, as if someone had drained the blood right out of my body.

I couldn't figure out why I was feeling so drained and so sad. My weight began to reach an all time high. I felt so embarrassed and didn't want to be seen in public, not even by my friends. "It's only a phase I'm going through, just snap out of it", I said to myself. I never did snap out of it. As a result, my weight jumped from 127 pounds to 158 pounds in just four months.

A Few Months Before the Diagnosis

I started noticing the nipple on my left breast wasn't as erect as it used to be. Even when I massaged the nipple it wouldn't become erect. In the past, when my body gave me warning signals I didn't want to listen, but now the warning signal was physically visible. I could see it with my own eyes. My gut feeling was telling me it was cancer. I didn't go to the doctor immediately because I was scared and hoped it would go away.

A few months passed and I noticed a puckering appear to the left of the same nipple. Now, I knew I was in trouble. Years ago I worked as the Director of Marketing for a mobile on-site mammography unit and I knew an inverted nipple and puckering were a strong indication of breast cancer (if you're saying to yourself, *"What a foolish girl"*, *you're absolutely right. All I can say to defend myself is that I wasn't ready for any more devastation in my life, so it was easier to ignore the symptoms).*

I called my primary care physician and scheduled an appointment. She examined my breasts and assured me it was nothing and I should just continue to watch it. So, I went home and continued watching it for one more month, during which time it got worse. I went to see her again. This time she prescribed a mammogram.

A few days later I received a call from her office with the results, *"Your mammogram is normal."* I knew deep within me the results were inaccurate.

Feeling frightened, I went back to my primary care physician. Holding firmly to her opinion she said, "I still think there's nothing wrong with your breast." At this point, I became frustrated and blurted out, *"If this was your breast, what would you do?"* Without hesitation she wrote out a prescription for me to see a surgeon.

A Few Weeks Before the Diagnosis

Finally, I was about to get down to the bottom of things. I made an appointment with the surgeon who my primary care physician recommended. All the way to the appointment I kept telling myself, "I'm fine, I'm going to be fine. It's going to be a cyst or something, not cancer."

During the examination, the surgeon felt confident it wasn't cancer. To be certain, she advised an ultra sound. I had the ultra sound that same week and during the procedure no signs of cancer were revealed. After the examination was completed the radiologist told me, that nine out of ten radiologists would not have recommended a needle biopsy based on my ultra sound results. In spite of this, her intuition told her to perform the biopsy just in case.

Two Days Before Cancer

On Wednesday July 9, 1997, I arrived at the mammography center for the needle biopsy. My friend Sharon, who I'm certain God personally appointed to be my angel here on earth, came with me. I was led into a small, but pleasant room with a table that had a hole cut out of it where my breast was to be placed. My knees began to shake and I desperately wanted to make a run for it.

Gently, the technician manipulated my body to be in perfect position for the biopsy. This wasn't as easy as it sounds. She had to readjust me several times before locking my breast in-between a vice! Lying face down on the table, with my breast squeezed in a vice for an hour, wasn't what I was anticipating. Most likely, physicians and surgeons don't tell us what to expect because they know we wouldn't show up!

What made this awful experience even remotely tolerable, was the radiologist telling me she would be surprised if the samples she was extracting were cancerous. She was almost positive they were not. I was so relieved and felt confident I didn't have cancer. Sharon and I celebrated the news by going out and enjoying a fabulous dinner.

Chapter Two

The Day I Received My Wake-up Call

On Friday July 11, 1997 at 2:30 in the afternoon, two days after the biopsy, I received my wake-up call. The same radiologist who performed the biopsy called and said, *"Agi, I've got some bad news. Your biopsy shows a carcinoma, breast cancer."*

My heart sank to a place so deep within my soul that had never been touched before. As we talked for a few more minutes, I sensed she was almost as shocked as I was. She even reiterated during our phone conversation that she really believed it wasn't cancer. "What do I do now?", I asked. She replied, "You have to see a surgeon as soon as possible." She gave me the name of a female surgeon who specializes in breast cancer surgery. "Let me know what happens", she said and we hung up the phone.

After a few minutes passed I thought, "What a rotten way to be told I have cancer." There's probably no good way to get this kind of devastating news, but when you're home alone it seems so heartless. Time somehow appeared

17

to stand still and my existence felt surreal. I remember walking around in circles saying, "I don't believe this, I don't believe this, I don't believe this." The phone call didn't seem real. One minute I was planning a romantic evening with Bill, and the next moment I was visualizing myself without a breast. *How could I have cancer, I was only thirty-eight years old?*

I became angry and shouted words I dare not write. A few minutes passed and I tried to be calm. I wasn't going to let cancer ruin my day. It didn't work. My heart jumped into my throat and I began to cry. I sat down on the bottom step of the staircase and continued to cry in disbelief.

Never in my entire life have I experienced the myriad of emotions as I did then. At first I was in disbelief, then I felt angry, after anger I felt sad and finally I went into shock.

I called Bill, and asked him to come home right away the biopsy results were in. I had cancer. He arrived home a half an hour later and found me sitting on the first step of the staircase, the same place I called him from. I must have sat there in shock and didn't move. As I heard him come through the garage, I didn't know whether to continue crying or to stop crying and be brave.

He rushed over and sat with me on the bottom step and held on to me for dear life. He comforted me in the most loving and tender way. With his love wrapped around me I felt so safe and secure.

My husband's thoughts on this devastating day.

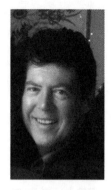

" When Agi called me, the brokenness in her voice created a numbness and sense of urgency in me. The weight of her words took effect. It was like getting punched in the stomach. You're without breath for a few moments.

All I wanted to do was comfort her,
love her and let her know everything
was going to be all right.

I found myself having a reaction on different levels including the physical, emotional, mental and spiritual. With some of the things that have happened to me in the past, the meaning of her words returned me to times and situations already been. As Yogi Berra said, "It's deja vu' all over again.

Even though in the past the situations were not cancer related they were nonetheless gut wrenching. This time there was not the shock that accompanied the life- changing day, my young daughter was hit by a car. She slipped into a coma and past away.

It was more like – I've been here before – It's ok – let's accept it and move with it. As the seriousness of the situation continued to wash over me, I found myself becoming stronger. Carrying hope and the knowledge that we would overcome this no matter how bad it appeared.

When I arrived home, Agi's response to the situation was going from one extreme to the other...and everywhere in between. At one moment, she would be angry, crying and the next, joking and laughing.

I listened held her close as she talked it out. It seems there's not a lot you can say at a time like this. You just have to receive it as the circumstances of the situation. Let it wash over you.

As we sat on the steps holding each other, we both seemed to reach a place of *peace*. It felt good to be quiet, both inside and out. All of a sudden, Agi jumped up and said, "Let's go out!" It felt like the right thing to do."

....After crying in his arms for a short while, an overwhelming strength came over me. I sprang to my feet, wiped away my tears and claimed victory over this cancer. I suggested we go out to dinner and get drunk. *(There was another reason I sprang to my feet and stopped crying. I'm not one to cry for long periods of time because my eyes get awfully swollen, my sinuses become congested and I look terrible the next day. My vanity took over and it got me to stop feeling devastated).*

We went to one of my favorite restaurants and I ordered peppered Ahi Tuna with a frozen margarita. It was strange, I couldn't taste the flavor of the Ahi Tuna or the margarita. My senses were numb along with the rest of me. I felt this feeling only one other time in my life and that was when my father and my sister died.

An indescribable feeling of 'KNOWING' swept over me. It's difficult to find the words to describe this feeling. The best way I know how to describe this knowing feeling is this...It's the *'without a shadow of a doubt' knowing that you know, that you know, that you know.* The knowing feeling that swept over me was of <u>DEATH</u>. I knew I was going to die, just as sure as I knew my name was Agi *(this was before I knew anything about natural healing).*

I also felt that cancer was somewhere else in my body, not only in my breast. At that moment, I related to the men, women and children aboard the sinking Titanic when they realized they had no chance for survival. Bill and I both agreed it was time to go home and comfort each other.

That evening as we held each other, Bill began to talk about God and how none of us are given more than we can handle.

During our conversation, I told Bill that I didn't blame God for the cancer in my body. I felt the cancer manifested as a result of the fear and anger I had experienced throughout my life.

While falling asleep in his arms, I had a strong urge to forgive all the people in my life who have ever wronged me in any way. I remember thinking, "I'll start tommorow."

Maryvale Samaritan
Medical Center

5102 West Campbell Avenue Phoenix, AZ 85031

ANATOMIC PATHOLOGY REPORT

MR# : (00883)137887
ACCT# : 0000000022851
NAME : BARBI, AGNEB

ADMIT: 07/10/97
DISCH: 07/10/97
REPORT PRINTED: 07/12/97   1700

AGE : 38 YRS   SEX : F
LOC : 07LAB   ROOM :

SOURCE OF TISSUE:
Left breast core biopsy.

CLINICAL DIAGNOSIS:
Asymmetric density, left breast, scarring vs fibrocystic change.

GROSS DESCRIPTION:
The specimen is received in formalin. It consists of elongated segments of
yellow and pink tissue measuring in aggregate up to 1.5 cm in length by 0.8 cm
in aggregate in diameter. The entire specimen is submitted in one
cassette.

MH :JB

MICROSCOPIC DESCRIPTION:
Sections show core biopsies of breast. The cores reveal an infiltrating
lobular carcinoma. Most of the cells are arranged in a single file. In other
areas small groups are formed. No tubular pattern is seen. Also, no lobular
carcinoma in situ or ductal carcinoma in situ is present in the sections.

PATHOLOGIC DIAGNOSIS:
Core biopsies of left breast, positive for infiltrating lobular carcinoma.

22

- Chapter Three -

The First Nine Days After My Wake-up Call

Surprisingly, the next morning on Saturday, July 12th, I woke up with a positive attitude. Determined to fight cancer and live to tell about it.

A few weeks before my wake-up call we had planned a party for that Saturday evening. Bill and I discussed canceling it, but after a very short discussion we decided to have the party. We needed to enjoy ourselves and *escape cancer for the evening.*

Several times throughout the day I went into the bathroom and stood in front of the mirror, just staring at my bare breasts. I'd cover my left breast and imagine what it would feel like when it was no longer there. I have to admit, I didn't care for the idea one bit.

What I haven't shared with you up until now, is that I had a breast augmentation, when I was thirty. For me, it wasn't about bigger breasts. It was about fixing deformed breasts that looked like they belonged to an eighty year- old woman.

For some reason, my breasts began deflating in my twenties. I had a complex about them and found myself obsessing over it. They looked liked Olive Oyl's breasts on the cartoon Popeye. So I did it and I'm glad I did. My self-esteem went through the roof and I was so happy.

In the afternoon, I took a few minutes to try to quite my mind. As I did, I began to see many of the people I harbored deep resentment and even hatred for. One by one, I visualized myself in front of them telling them I forgive them for hurting, disappointing or deceiving me.

It was 7:30 that Saturday evening and our friends were arriving for the party. By this time most of them knew about the cancer and were prepared to see me. We exchanged heart-felt hugs, talked a bit about my situation and then proceeded to have fun, just like old times. We danced and laughed for the next six hours. At about 2:30 in the morning, I announced that I was pooped out and the party was over.

After everyone left, a profound feeling of sadness came upon me and I felt so alone. The reality of having cancer in my body hit me like a Mack truck.

I wanted to call my mother, but I couldn't bring myself to do it. So instead, with a heavy heart and a drained spirit I went upstairs and fell asleep.

Second Day

The next day Sunday, July 13th was difficult. Again I wrestled with whether or not to call my mother. I picked up the phone several times throughout the day, but never dialed the number. The fact that her daughter had cancer would devastate her and I didn't want to be responsible for that. As you already know, my mother lost her only son to a drowning accident. I knew she would fall apart.

I might have told her I had cancer the day I found out, if we had relatives close by that could stay with her and comfort her, but we didn't.

Most of my day was spent talking to my friends and walking around in circles, not accomplishing much of anything. Later that evening, Sharon called and told me about a book she had recently read. The book was about healing herbs. In the book were actual cases about people who were healed from all sorts of life threatening diseases.

Sharon also read about Red Clover Tea and how effective it was in cleansing the blood. It all sounded promising. After her phone call, I decided to start making changes in my own lifestyle. *It's a shame it took cancer to get me to eat healthy.*

Third Day

On Monday, July 14th, I met again with the surgeon who recommended the ultra sound, which led to the biopsy. As I walked up to the window to sign in I felt like everyone in the waiting room knew I had cancer. I signed in and was immediately escorted into the examination room.

A few minutes later the surgeon came in. She was sympathetic to my situation and as gently as she could, she advised me to have a radical mastectomy, removal of certain lymph nodes and chemotherapy. A cold chill ran down my spine and I tried not to cry. "Be strong Agi, be strong", I said to myself. All of a sudden, I heard myself agreeing to the mastectomy. It didn't seem real and I began to feel sick to my stomach. The room seemed to be getting smaller and smaller. *All I could think about was getting out of there.*

The surgeon handed me a prescription to see a re-constructive plastic surgeon and said she would hold me up in prayer at her next church meeting. I thanked her for keeping me in her prayers and told her I would call her office after I met with the plastic surgeon.

Fourth Day

The following morning on Tuesday, July 15th, I went for the standard blood work required before surgery. On my way home I felt a sudden urge to drive to an herb store. I remembered seeing one just a few blocks away and without any hesitation drove to the store. Once inside, I felt like a kid in a candy store. There were so many containers filled with leaves, roots, flowers, seeds, teas and herbal formulas. It was so new and exciting. This was my first experience with herbal remedies.

I began sharing my situation with the store clerk and told her about the upcoming surgery. Remembering what

Sharon said about Red Clover Tea, I asked the clerk if she had any of this tea. Before I could get the answer, a man in his 30's, named Larry, purchasing a large quantity of herbs turned to me and proclaimed, *"You don't need surgery."* Well, let me tell you, he got my attention. He proceeded to tell me about natural alternatives to surgery.

Later that evening Bill and I drove to Larry's home where he gave us 300 pages of the most incredible natural remedies as described by Dr. Richard Schulze. Driving home with the 300 pages in my lap, I knew the answer to my healing was somewhere inside.

The minute we arrived home, I began reading and didn't stop until finishing all 300 pages. "This is my new found hope", I thought with confidence.

Inside this treasure were stories about people who were healed naturally, from all sorts of life threatening diseases, mostly by cleansing their bodies and juice fasting. One man with leukemia had undergone different treatments and chemotherapy. He couldn't imagine any more chemotherapy treatments. Dr. Schulze started him on the "Incurables Program" immediately.

This man with leukemia started juice fasting and following the program faithfully. The first month he didn't improve, so he took a break for a week and ate only raw foods. He then went back on juicing for another month. Some of his blood counts were coming up and he was stabilizing. Once again he went back on raw foods for a while before beginning the third month of juicing. That's when big changes were seen. His blood chemistry began changing dramatically. By the fifth month he was cancer free.

Another case I read about involved a young twenty-three year old woman who had a malignant tumor in her left breast (just like me). Her doctor wanted to schedule her for a mastectomy, but first she went to see Dr. Schulze.

She went to work immediately juicing, cleansing her body and applying poultices on her breast (a poultice is made by mixing herbs with either water or oil until it reaches the consistency of a paste. In this case, it was a poultice of herbs that would penetrate into the breast and attack cancer).

Within seven days she could hardly feel the lump. She went back to the doctor and was told it was reduced by 50%. She was so excited, went home and worked even harder. Ten days later, she went back for another check up and the doctor could find **NO signs of cancer in her breast.**

"So why couldn't I be one of these people and what makes them any different than me?", played over and over and over in my mind while I read about these cases. After finishing all 300 pages I knew, without a shadow of a doubt, that *natural healing was the path for me* to follow. An overwhelming heaviness was lifted off of my spirit. The excitement and challenge of cleansing my body and killing this cancer began to energize me. I could hardly wait to get started.

Fifth Day

On Wednesday morning, July 16th, I woke up feeling tremendously empowered. I was anxious to get a juicer and start juicing fresh organic vegetables.

For some reason, I still kept my appointment with the plastic surgeon that day. All the way to his office I asked myself, "Why am I doing this? I know I'm not going to have surgery."

When I arrived, a friendly assistant led me to an examination room and gave me the standard gown with the opening in the front. The room was freezing cold and I felt so uneasy being there. Reluctantly, I put the gown on and waited for twenty minutes before the surgeon came in. I was quickly becoming aggravated and annoyed. I began to ask him questions about the procedure and about his experience with re-constructive surgery. With confidence he replied, "I'm great at what I do."

He then proceeded to examine my breasts and rather arrogantly began to tell me they were too saggy. He could make them look perky again (one of the reasons I love my breasts so much is that they don't look augmented. I'll admit it, they do sag a little, but that's what makes them look real). *If I let him have his way, today I'd be appearing on the talk show circuit with the first reconstructed breasts coming out of my chin!*

I'm sure he thought he was making me feel better, but instead I was offended and wanted to *punch him in the nose!*

He sat down in a chair next to the examination table, where I was sitting, and gave me a photo album to look through. The album was filled with pictures of former re-constructive patients of his. As I was looking through the photos, out of the corner of my eye, I noticed that he had taken off his shoe and had begun to scratch his foot. Not just a little scratch... he was so into it that the building could have been on fire and he wouldn't have stopped scratching.

Utterly grossed out I thought, "This guy is disgusting and probably has athletes foot. I don't want him anywhere near my breasts." I tried not to stare and bit my tongue (which is very rare for me to do) as I hurried through the photo album. At last, he stopped scratching and asked me if I had any further questions. I didn't and hoped he wouldn't try to shake my hand goodbye. Luckily he didn't.

This was the final confirmation I was given. I knew I was making the right decision choosing natural healing.

The minute I got home, I called the radiologist, the surgeon, the re-constructive surgeon and my primary care physician. I informed them that I had changed my mind. Both the radiologist and the surgeon advised against natural healing and graciously wished me well.

Appallingly, my primary care physician (a woman nevertheless) told me point blank, *"I think your decision is STUPID."* This is the same physician who told me there was nothing wrong with my breast even when my nipple was inverting and had puckering next to it. Needless to say, she's no longer my primary care physician.

Last but not least, I left a message at the reconstructive surgeon's office. Trying to control myself from laughing, I asked the office manager to inform the doctor that he was disgusting and needed to have his athlete foot looked at! She giggled and said she would make sure he got the message.

Feeling confident about my decision, I phoned Larry to tell him that I had chosen 'The Incurables Program' to heal my body. As we got deeper into conversation, I was beginning to realize the enormous amount of work ahead of me. The Incurables Program would take ten to fourteen hours a day of continually preparing, juicing, drinking teas, taking herbal formulas, hot cold therapy and more.

I began to feel overwhelmed and wondered if I had made the right decision. If I knew even the slightest bit about juicing or herbal remedies or even how to brew tea, it may not have been so overwhelming. Larry gave me the phone number of a man in North Carolina who was familiar with the Incurables Program and would help me get started.

Ending my conversation with Larry, I immediately called this man. His name is Charles, and he began to share his knowledge of the Program. He went on to tell me about people he knew who had completely healed from life threatening diseases, following this natural healing program.

About ten minutes into our conversation I told him I didn't think I could do this all on my own and needed help. He gave me the phone number of a woman, named Mary Ann, who lived in California and facilitated cleansing programs.

Thanking Charles for his help, I hung up the phone and called Mary Ann. A sweet angelic voice answered the phone. Enthusiastically, I began to explain my situation and how I needed help to get started on my journey to natural healing. Mary Ann began to tell me about the natural health program she facilitates at CedarBrook. She described a serene setting where I would learn about God's Laws of Natural Health and the basic principles of cleansing the body. I responded by blurting out, "Great, when can I come?" With compassion Mary Ann replied, "I don't have room for you this month, but I do next month in August you can come then."

My heart dropped to floor and in desperation I replied, *"If I don't come this month I'll give in and go through with the surgery.* Please, please is there anyway I can come?" Mary Ann replied, "Let me see what I can do, but I can't promise anything." She said she would call me if it were at all possible.

Before ending our conversation I asked if there was anything I could do to prepare for my stay (positive thinking). Mary Ann suggested I begin to juice and eat live foods. I thanked her for her kindness and begged her again to make room for me. I told her I'd sleep on the floor if I had to. After hanging up the phone, I prayed and prayed someone would cancel so I could go.

Sixth Day

The next day on Thursday, July 17th, the first thing I did was to purchase a juicer. I then bought some organic carrots, apples, celery and parsley and began to juice. By preparing fresh juice, I was becoming proactive in my own healing. This gave me a renewed sense of empowerment.

Mary Ann called back that afternoon and said, *"Pack your bags and be here Sunday, July 20th, by noon."* I was so excited. After thanking her endless times, I began jumping with joy shouting, "Yahoo, Yahoo!"

I phoned Bill at work and gave him the good news. He immediately arranged my airline reservations. That evening Bill and I rejoiced and praised God, for we knew it was His doing.

Seventh Day

Finally on Friday, July 18th, I phoned my mother and told her I had cancer. Just as I thought, she fell apart and began to cry. I explained to her what I knew about natural healing and told her I was going to CedarBrook. There I would learn more about natural healing and how to cleanse my body. This just fueled the fire because she just couldn't understand how I could choose natural healing over traditional medicine.

After going around and around with her and getting nowhere, I became stern and told her what I needed was support in my decision, not opposition. If she couldn't be supportive I wouldn't see her until I was healed.

I know this sounds really harsh and you may be thinking, "How could she speak to her mother that way?" You must understand that at this point, even though my mind was made up and I chose natural healing, I was still riding a fine line between being confident about my decision and doubting my decision.

So for me, to hear my mother's doubt and disapproval could very easily have caused me to change my mind. The only way I knew of to stay focused and on my journey was to respond to her the way I did.

Later that same day, shortly after having spoken with my mother, the radiologist and surgeon's office called once more trying to talk me into having surgery, as soon as possible. Holding steadfast, *I told them I wouldn't change my mind and to please stop calling me.*

I couldn't wait for Sunday to come so I could escape and begin my healing journey.

As the hours went by, I began to teeter-totter on my decision again. Bill and I spent time talking about the decision and the events leading up to it. He reassured me that he believed it was the right decision and that God would continue to guide us through this.

By this time, I experienced withdrawal symptoms from caffeine and sugar. For the past few days, I only juiced fresh vegetables and ate a few pieces of fruit. My head hurt continuously all day. I looked terrible and felt awful.

My friends told me some months after that they were really worried about me and questioned my decision.

Eighth Day

Saturday evening, July 19th, was the turning point in my life. Lou and his wife Sharon (my dear friend) arrived at our home at 8:00 p.m. After we exchanged hugs and kisses, all four of us sat down at the dining room table. We held hands and gave thanks for our friendship.

Then Lou, Sharon and Bill began to pray for my safe trip to CedarBrook and the successful cleansing of my body. As they were praying, I felt a vibration fill the inside of my body and I saw a beautiful golden light surround me. It was a sensation I've never felt before. I felt peaceful, exhilarated, and completely open all at the same time.

When I first met Bill I remember saying to him, "Just because you believe in God doesn't mean I have too, right?" Bill and I began talking about God more often after my brother died, but I never would have imagined I would ever experience what I did that evening.

Ninth Day

On Sunday morning, July 20th, I woke up feeling wonderful considering I only had four hours of sleep. With bags packed, I was ready to go and begin my healing journey.

"Life
and the art
of living it,
is not in
the arrival
or
departure
but in the
journey"

Chapter Four

My Initiation...
Into A Healthy Lifestyle

On Sunday evening, July 20th, I arrived at CedarBrook, nestled peacefully in the mountains of Northern California. Mary Ann graciously welcomed me in. Within minutes it felt like I was at home. That evening, I met the others who were about to embark on the same adventure I was. We enjoyed a deliciously healthy dinner and discussed what to expect in the days to come.

After dinner, I took a moment to listen to the sounds of the whispering pines and breathe in the fresh air. It felt so right for me to be there.

The following nine days were filled learning about and experiencing God's Eight Laws of Natural Health, which are: *Pure air, sunlight, abstemiousness, rest, exercise, proper diet, the use of water and trust in divine power.*

Each day a different cleansing process took place involving either my colon, liver, gall bladder, kidneys, blood or skin.

The first morning, I sprang out of bed with eagerness to begin the day. We all greeted each other, recorded our blood pressure and pulse. Then we began the cleansing process by drinking one-half gallon of isotonic sea-water. It was awful. I thought, "This must be my personal initiation into natural healing."

Why couldn't this cleanse begin with something sweet? Struggling to drink the water, I seriously contemplated packing my bags and going home.

The first two mornings were rough. I couldn't bear to drink any more isotonic water without the help of a lemon or slice of lime. After I quit my moaning and groaning the rest of the day seemed easy.

By the third day we were all anxious to eat real food. We fantasized about pizza, pasta, anything. What we soon came to realize was that *real food was fresh live fruits, vegetables, nuts, seeds and whole grains.*

To my surprise, I found myself enjoying these live foods. Who would ever have thought? Any doubt of my healing completely vanished. This is the support system I needed to be a part of.

My headache lessoned with each day of cleansing. By the fourth day I felt terrific.

Each morning before getting out of bed, I thanked God for enabling me to come to CedarBrook. I then asked for a word for the day *(I'm not sure who first said the quote, "never say never", but he or she was a wise person. Years ago, if someone were to predict that I would be reading the Bible first thing in the morning, my response to them would have been a rude one).*

Nevertheless, there I was snuggled up in my bed, looking out my bedroom window into the woods, and opening randomly to a page in the New Testament. I consistently received the following reading:

Matthew 9:20-22
Cure of the woman with a hemorrhage.

"Then from behind him came a woman, who had suffered from a hemorrhage for twelve years, and she touched the fringe of his cloak, for she said to herself, "If I can only touch his cloak I shall be well again." Jesus turned around and saw her and he said to her, "Courage, my daughter, your faith had restored you to health." And from that moment the woman was well again."

The message I personally received from this reading was of unquestionable and undoubting faith. Faith and healing went hand in hand. In order for me to receive complete healing, I needed to have undoubting and unfaltering faith.

This picture was taken one year before I was diagnosed with breast cancer.

I was out of control and falling into a depression. I weighed over 152 pounds and food became my comfort.

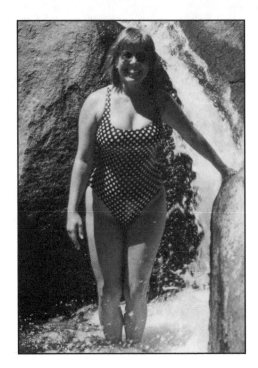

I weighed 140 pounds when I first arrived at CedarBrook. After nine days of cleansing my body with fresh squeezed vegetable and fruit juices, I weighed 131 pounds. I felt fantastic and full of energy. My entire outlook on food changed dramatically. *No longer did I crave meat and sweets. Instead, I craved fresh live foods that would build my health. I wanted to live!*

Leaving was difficult and very emotional. Saying goodbye to my fellow cleansing group and the staff, especially Mary Ann, was hard. I wanted to go home, pack up all of my belongings, come back and never leave.

- Chapter *Five* -

The Incurables Program

After coming home from CedarBrook, I started on this program and stayed on it for six weeks. The Incurables Program is an intensive cleansing program. Dr. Schulze designed the Incurables Program for his patients who were diagnosed with incurable diseases. The program consists of juicing fresh vegetables for one month (or longer if necessary), cleansing the entire body, hydrotherapy, exercise, deep breathing exercises, maintaining the "I can do it" attitude, and no eating cooked foods.

At CedarBrook, we viewed videotapes of Dr. Schulze explaining the Incurables Program during one of his Healing Crusade Seminars. As I listened to his testimonies and aggressive approach to natural healing, I found myself agreeing with what he was saying. *He believes the body is capable of healing itself when given the proper tools.*

Both of Dr. Schulze's parents died from heart attacks by the time they were 55 years old. At 16 years of age he was diagnosed with an incurable genetic heart deformity. He was told he would only live to be 20 years old. By changing his lifestyle his heart healed naturally. Since then, his mission has been to help others beat the odds.

For over twenty years Dr. Schulze operated a clinic, first in New York and later moving it to Southern California. He witnessed thousands of his clients heal from life threatening illnesses. Authorities dismissed these healings and insisted Dr. Schulze was practicing medicine without a license.

Although Dr. Schulze holds a Doctorate of Herbology, a Doctorate in Natural Medicine, a degree in Herbal Pharmacy and degrees in Iridology, authorities have dismissed his successes and insisted he cease practicing. Coming close to being imprisoned numerous times gave him no alternative, but to close his practice and begin to share his knowledge and experience with others through his world-wide seminars.

Dr. Schulze is considered to be an innovator, even an extremist by many of his colleagues, but to his clients he was considered, "The man who has the guts to say and do what others were afraid to."

Everyone who knows me will tell you the same thing about me. I knew I had to be aggressive with the cancer still in my body and I knew by following the Incurables Program, I was going to kill it. Never in my wildest dreams did I think I would see cancer be expelled from my body! Yes, you read it right. *As God is my witness, I saw with my own eyes what cancer looks like. I'll give full details in the Cold Sheet Treatment chapter.*

An In-depth Look at The Incurables Program

The Food Program

For six weeks, I never allowed a piece of cooked food to enter my mouth. Instead, twice a day I drank a super nutrition green drink, which is a natural source of vitamins and minerals. In addition, I drank six glasses of freshly juiced carrots with apples, parsley, celery, and ginger root.

After a week of the same juices, I ventured out and began juicing spinach, lettuce and whatever else was green. I also drank one gallon of distilled water each day.

My weight dropped from around 131 pounds to 110 pounds after one month of juicing. My friends thought I was going to wither away to skin and bones. They were beginning to get worried.

I had to constantly reinforce to them the knowledge I had acquired which was: **In order for me to achieve complete healing my body had to continue cleansing until it was completely clean** (which meant it may have to get down to skin and bones). My body knew how much weight it could lose before it would build itself back up again.

I wasn't afraid. I had complete faith in what I was doing. Even though I looked shallow and very skinny, I had great color in my face and FELT GREAT! My energy level was sky high and my thinking was clearer than it has ever been in my entire life!

Symptoms of Tourette's syndrome were even going away. My allergies were completely gone and best of all, my knees felt brand new. For years I've suffered with chronic knee problems. At least once a month, for the past two years before starting on this program, I had to ice my knees to keep the swelling down. I couldn't play tennis or go hiking without a knee brace.

I'm convinced that eliminating meat, dairy, sugar and flour products for the entire month enabled my knees to be fully restored to perfect condition.

O.K. so I'd like to say the entire month of juicing was a breeze, but it wasn't. I'd say 85% of the time I felt strong and vibrant. While 15% of the time I felt deprived of the foods I was used to. The blood cleanse was the hardest for me to do. During the five days of blood cleansing I felt spaced out and fatigued. Drinking carrot juice started to gag me, and by the third week, I never wanted to drink carrot juice as long as I lived.

I consumed **3-6 cloves of fresh raw garlic** everyday. Garlic is one of the most potent and reliable herbal healers known. It's a powerful broad spectrum antibiotic, anti-viral, anti-fungal and anti-parasitic, and has been proven to rid the body internally and externally of any antigens or pathogens. My friends had a hard time being around me!

Potassium Broth helped flush toxins, poisons, unwanted salts and acids out of my system, while at the same time, my body was receiving vitamins and minerals. I made a large pot every week.

Recipe:

- ✓ Fill a large pot with organic: ¼ potato peelings, ¼ carrot peelings and one beet chopped (optional), 1/2 chopped onions, 4-5 stalks of celery cut in half, dark greens like; spinach, kale, chard, mustard greens and parsley, and at least 20-50 garlic cloves. Add hot peppers or jalapeno to spice it up, if you like.
- ✓ Add enough distilled water to cover vegetables and simmer on low, for 1-2 hours (never bring to a boil)
- ✓ Strain and drink only the broth

This is a potent vitamin and mineral drink. I still make it today, especially during the flu season.

Intestinal Cleansing Program was
extremely important during this program. With the help of: Cascara Sagrada, Barberry Rootbark, Ginger, Garlic and African Bird Pepper I was able to keep the toxins expelling from my body.

Cleansing the Liver and Gallbladder
helped me rebuild my liver, which was damaged from hepatitis. Some of the herbs used for doing this were: Milk Thistle, Dandelion, Oregon Grape Root, Wormwood, Black Walnut Hulls, Ginger, Garlic and Sweet Fennel Seed.

First thing in the morning, for five days I mixed the following ingredients to help cleanse my liver and gall bladder:

- ✓ 8 ounces of fresh orange juice
- ✓ 1-5 cloves of garlic (started with one and increased to five)
- ✓ 1-5 tablespoons of organic virgin cold-pressed olive oil (started with one increased to five)
- ✓ 1 piece of ginger root (about an inch long)

15 minutes after drinking this concoction, I consumed a Detoxification Herb Tea which had Dandelion Root, Pau d'Arco, Cinnamon, Cardamon, Licorice, Fennel, Juniper Berries, Ginger, Clove, Uva Ursi, Parsley Root and a few more hers. With this tea I drank 2 dropperfuls of a Liver/Gall Bladder & and Anti-Parasite Formulae. I repeated this tea mixture two more times each day.

Kidney and Bladder Cleanse was beneficial for my kidneys and my bladder since I've had problems with both.

First thing in the morning, for five days I mixed:

- ✓ the juice of one lemon and one lime
- ✓ 16-32 ounces of distilled water
- ✓ a big pinch of Cayenne powder
- ✓ 15 minutes after this lip-smacking eye opening drink, I consumed 2 cups of the Kidney/Bladder-Dissolve Tea. Some of the herbs in this tea are: Uva Ursi, Juniper Berries, Corn silk, Horsetail Herb, Burdock Root, Pipsissewa Leaf. 2 dropperfuls of Kidney/Bladder Formula. I repeated this tea mixture two more times each day.

The Blood and Lymphatic Cleanse was

intense. During the second and third week I consumed 4 ounces of this formula each week, which equaled 2 dropperfuls, 4-6 times a day. My blood must have been so toxic and polluted that I literally babbled the first day. My words were slurred and what I was thinking wasn't coming out of my mouth. I know this sounds scary but I wasn't afraid because I'd been learning about the blood cleanse before I did it. Some of the blood cleansing herbs are: Red Clover Blossoms, Chaparral, Poke Root, Oregon Grape Root, Burdock Root and Seed, Yellow Dock and Bloodroot.

Building the Immune System was vital in

my healing. During the second and fourth week I consumed 4 ounces of Echinacea. *Are you beginning to see how much work I had to do in one day? It turned into a 12-14 hour a day job.*

The Hydrotherapy Program took some

doing. At the time I didn't belong to a health club to enjoy the benefits of a steam sauna. Also, it was summertime and in Arizona we have NO cold water to easily do the hot and cold showers. So here's what I did: I loaded up bowls of ice and took them into the shower with me. I stood under very hot water for a minute then poured ice water over my entire body. Repeating this process three times, every day and some nights. The goal of hot and cold showers is to stimulate the blood flow and get it moving.

I did a **high enema each week** for four weeks even though I felt extremely cleansed by now. Each enema was followed by an implant enema consisting of: 16 ounces of distilled water, 1 capsule of acidophilus to replace friendly bacteria and 2ozs of wheat grass.

I brushed my skin every day, with a dry natural plant-fiber skin-brush. I started at my feet and moved upward toward my heart, paying special attention to my breasts, lymphatic system, my thigh area and under my arms.

I ran, hiked or roller bladed for one hour every day. I bounced on a mini trampoline because it's an effective way to get the lymphatic system stimulated.

Deep Breathing oxygenates the blood and stimulates the lymphatic and circulation systems. I did deep breathing exercises 3-4 times each day (and still do).

I take a deep breath in through my nose and hold it for 4 counts. Then I exhaled slowly through my mouth to the count of 10, repeating this process 4-5 times.

Additional Healing Tips:

♦ Everyday, I took a sun-bath for 10 to 15 minutes
♦ Everyday, I took a walk barefoot in the grass
♦ Used only natural soaps, toothpaste and deodorant
♦ Thanked God for my life every morning, noon and night

Please read: If you are considering doing The Incurables Program please, consult your physician or a qualified health practitioner so that they can monitor you along the way. This natural treatment is very beneficial. It can also be very dangerous if not followed precisely.

Chapter Six

The Cold Sheet Treatment

_____

The Cold Sheet Treatment is included in the Incurables Program. It's a method of using hot and cold hydrotherapy to increase the activity of the immune cells, which in turn fight disease.

This treatment can accelerate the speed of your white blood cells by up to 64 times. When the immune system is stimulated to this level, infections and even cancer can be destroyed. "Most people don't realize it, but with the Cold Sheet Treatment, we are using a principle of medicine called leuco-taxis", explains Dr. Schulze. This is where the activity and motion of white blood cells increase in response to heat." I watched a video tape where Dr. Schulze was helping a woman through the cold sheet treatment. I was nervous but decided this was the next step in my healing.

My Experience...
With The Cold Sheet Treatment.

I experienced my first Cold Sheet Treatment two weeks after finishing the Incurables Program. It was Sunday morning on September 14th, Bill, Sharon and Linda were about to be initiated into the "Cold Sheet Club." My friend Michal became a member of the club during my third Cold Sheet Treatment.

Eagerly, yet nervously, I prepared the dishtowel filled with a handful of powdered cayenne, ginger and mustard seed powder. Already my sinuses were being cleansed from all the sneezing I was doing, due to the potency of the herbs in the air. Next, I began to brew the six cups of yarrow and peppermint tea. At this point tension was beginning to build...I couldn't believe I was going through with it!

Moving right along, I peeled eight cloves of organic garlic and placed it in the blender with ½ cup of raw apple cider vinegar and ½ cup of distilled water. I set the blender on chop for a minute and it did the job. Little did I know my rear end was about to feel the same way the garlic did being chopped up in the blender.

The "Cold Sheet Club" arrived and cheered me on. Bill put on peaceful music to keep the atmosphere calm, as we were about to embark on an adventure of enormous faith and courage. We said a prayer asking God to be with us and to guide us through this process.

My heart raced as I held the enema bag filled with garlic. I asked Bill to stay around the corner of the bedroom, just in case. I closed the bathroom doors and injected the garlic enema. Not more than 15 seconds passed when I jumped up, let out a yelp, and rushed to get this stuff out.

Dr. Schulze was right, he described it as a Napalm Bomb going off in your rear end. I thought, "What was I doing, was it worth this pain?" I didn't know whether to cry or laugh, so I did both.

After a few minutes, the cramping subsided. I regained my composure, got brave and looked into the toilet. OOH, YUK....it looked like a handful of tubular whitish, fleshy, tissue stuff. I thought it was worms that had died from the garlic and fell out of me. I know now (from my herbalist schooling) that it was mucus and candida being expelled from my body. I heard Bill shouting, "Are you all right, are you all right?" I'm sure the others were downstairs wondering what they got themselves into and should they stay or go?

About four to five minutes later, my knees regained their strength. "O.K. Agi, you got through that part and it wasn't too bad. Just keep going", I reassured myself. I proceeded to put Vaseline over my private parts and my nipples. I used half a jar to protect them from being burnt from the herbs in the water.

The "Cold Sheet Club" then joined me as I stepped slowly into the bathtub and cautiously sat down. (The bathtub was filled with very hot water, as hot as I could stand). I began squeezing the dishtowel with the herbs in it (to get more of the herbs in the water). To my surprise, a big clump of the herbs escaped out of the dishtowel and into my bath water!

Bill quickly grabbed the "not" so tightly wrapped dishtowel and threw it in the sink. The water was a yellowish brown. We couldn't even see through it. We all started sneezing and our eyes began to water. It was funny, we burst into laughter. We all needed a good laugh at that point.

Within the first few minutes, I drank my first cup of hot peppermint tea. Bill asked me how I was feeling. I told him I didn't feel the heat yet. After 10 minutes, sweat started beading up on my forehead and my skin was beginning to feel the burning of the cayenne, mustard seed and ginger in the water.

Bill handed me another cup of tea, while Linda and Sharon cheered me on. My skin was really starting to burn and I could feel my fever rising. The next three cups of tea were harder to drink and I was beginning to feel a little weak. Bill wiped my forehead with a *cold wet hand-towel and let it rest on top of my head.* He refreshed the hand-towel several times for the duration of the bath.

Sweat was pouring down my face, but I only had five minutes left to reach my goal of thirty minutes. The last cup of tea almost didn't make it down. Finally, thirty minutes passed and I couldn't wait to get out! I felt weak and needed help getting out of the tub. I had a fever, but my body didn't ache like it has in the past from fevers related to colds and flu.

Bill helped me out of the tub and wrapped a king size cold sheet, *that's been soaking in ice water for an hour before I got into the bath,* around me. **WOW!** The first second was a shock and then the ice-cold sheet was a welcomed relief from the heat. Wrapped up like a mummy, they put me to bed and covered me up with a comforter (the bed was protected with a plastic cover under the sheets, so was my pillow).

Almost immediately, I asked for some room temperature distilled water. I was kind of paranoid about drinking enough fluids, so I made sure I did. I couldn't unwrap my arms, so Bill kind of pushed me up from my back and Linda put the straw up to my lips so I could drink.

Sharon continuously wiped my eyes with a hand-towel because my face was pouring water like an open faucet. My legs and arms felt like someone was putting a hot iron on them. It was on the verge of being painful, but it never got unbearable. I'm sure the burning feeling was from the herbs falling out of the towel into the water and getting on my skin (this little accident turned out to be beneficial, because I believe it helped raise my temperature more than if they hadn't spilled out).

After twenty minutes being wrapped in the cold sheet, my entire body felt like a water faucet left turned on. Water was literally pouring out of my face, arms and legs. We didn't take my temperature, although everyone agreed it must have been 103 or 104 degrees. The fever broke about an hour later. I managed to stay wrapped in the sheet for another hour. I knew it was best to stay in the sheet all night, but I couldn't do it.

After two hours of intense sweating, I felt weak but clear minded. All in all, I felt really great considering what my body just went through. An urgency to go to the bathroom came upon me. I unwrapped myself and slowly walked into the bathroom. My legs were a little shaky.

My curiosity got to me and I looked into the toilet. A handful of the same fleshy, whitish, tubular fuzzy stuff came out, as did with the garlic enema. Still thinking they were worms, I felt relieved knowing they were coming out of me instead of growing inside of me.

I began to think back to the times in Mexico when I would eat from the vendors on the streets. "This is where these worms must of come from. I'll never eat food from street carts again", I vowed.

Moving very slowly, I stepped into the shower and washed my entire body, even my hair, with raw apple cider vinegar.

After the shower I changed into warm clothes and joined the "Cold Sheet Club" downstairs.

We discussed the experience we all just shared. They were anxious to hear what came out of me. At the same time they were grossed out, wondering what must be inside of them.

A few hours later, the "The Cold Sheet Club" went home. Shortly after they left, I began to develop a sinus headache that quickly turned into a sinus infection. I immediately picked up a book on natural healing and found the section related to sinuses. I read about an herbal remedy using ginger powder to help clear the sinuses. I went right to work.

First, I rinsed my sinuses with a solution of warm water and sea salt. Then I made a paste by mixing ginger powder and water. I applied this mixture to my sinus area for ten minutes. After washing it off, the pain from the infection seemed to subside. I repeated this process one more time that day and then went to bed.

The next day the sinus infection was gone, but I still felt a little weak. I realized why I developed the sinus. *I didn't elevate my head during the Cold Sheet Treatment.* As the day went by I began to regain my strength. By the following morning *I felt like I was sixteen years old again!*

My Incredible Experience After The Second Cold Sheet Treatment

One week after my first Cold Sheet Treatment I was ready to do the second one. I followed the same steps as the first time, but this time I made sure the dishtowel with the herbs in it was better secured. We also put towels under my head and feet to elevate them. I blew my nose more often to insure I wouldn't get another sinus infection.

My fever didn't seem as high this time. We all guessed the fever to be about 101-102 degrees. After two hours of being wrapped in the cold sheet, I had the urgency to go to the bathroom.

This time it wasn't the whitish, fleshy, tubular wormy looking stuff. Instead it was **a long piece of tar-like sea-weedy rope; about 6 inches long with three white fuzzy egg-like objects attached to it.** YUK! This really grossed me out.

At CedarBrook I looked through a book that had pictures of the same sea-weed-like stuff in it. Knowing what it was kept me from freaking out. I knew this seaweed-like stuff was the oldest and most toxic poisonous material lodged deep inside my colon. There weren't any pictures of the white eggs, so what were they?

The "Cold Sheet Club" was anxiously waiting to hear what came out of me this time. I climbed back into bed and they came running in to hear the details. Not more than two minutes passed when I scooted them all back out again so I could return to the bathroom.

This time the only thing that fell out of me was an object the size of a half-dollar. Nothing else came out. No fecal matter, no seaweed-like stuff, nothing but this thing!

It was the color of flesh with a tiny bit of brown in it, round with three legs on one side and three legs on the other side. It had a little brownish black round ball that looked like the head. It looked just like a CRAB!

Yuk, YUK, YUK, I was completely disgusted. I thought this was mama parasite coming out and the long green seaweed looking thing with the eggs on it were her kids, getting ready to hatch, AUH!

I was prepared to save a sample of whatever came out of me this time so I could get it analyzed. Holding a plastic cup and long spoon, I reached in to try to get it, but it kept slipping off the spoon. After a few more attempts I knew I couldn't save it, so I flushed it down the toilet.

After my apple cider vinegar shower we all discussed what in the world this crab could have been. The "Cold Sheet Club" was even more concerned now about what must be in their bodies. After about a half an hour of speculating, I went upstairs and went to bed. The next morning I felt great! The whole inside of my body was renewed and refreshed. It's difficult to put into words how I felt. *I was so clear. More clear than I've ever been in my entire life.* My body felt new, without any disease or discomfort.

A few days after expelling this crab-like thing, I went to the library to see if I could find out what it was. I couldn't find any information, absolutely nothing. So instead, I decided to read up on the Lobular Carcinoma I was diagnosed with. I found a book, which described the different types of breast cancer. My stomach began to get uptight as I proceeded to read the prognosis for different types of breast cancer.

The prognosis for some were excellent, for others good, for others fair and for the carcinoma I had the prognosis was poor. Ouch! I got a bad feeling in the pit of my stomach that I couldn't shake for most of the day. I kept reminding myself that I was getting a full healing.

I asked God to take these thoughts from my mind and to give me the strength to keep my faith. The next day was better and a few days later, I stopped thinking about it all together.

The second Cold Sheet Treatment was the highlight of them all. Nothing else gruesome came out of me during the third and fourth treatments, but a tiny bit more of what I thought were worms (knowing now it was mucus and probably more candida).

During the fourth Cold Sheet Treatment, my temperature didn't seem to get as high and I was only wrapped up in the cold sheet for 1½ hours

Several months later, while I was doing a homework assignment, for my schooling to become an herbalist, I read about a woman who expelled the same kind of crab-like thing from her body. She expelled it six months after following a program similar to the one I was on.

I don't know how she managed to save it, but she did. She took the crab-like thing to the pathologist and was told it was spider cancer. I was ecstatic after reading her testimony. At that point, I knew the crab-like creature that I expelled from my bowels was indeed spider cancer.

* *I must have had cancer in my colon or stomach. Not only in my breast.*

An illustration of what came out of me, after the second Cold Sheet Treatment.

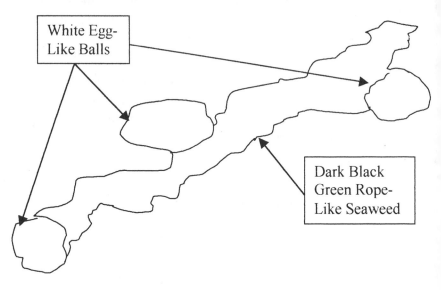

White Egg-Like Balls

Dark Black Green Rope-Like Seaweed

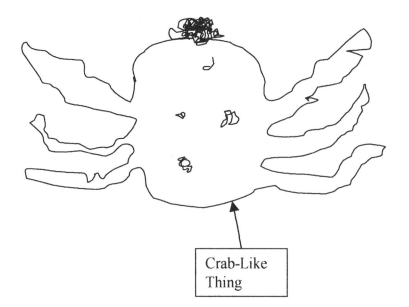

Crab-Like Thing

Chapter Seven

My Healing Diet the First Year

After completing the Incurables Program, I chose to continue on my healing journey following Dr. Christopher's Mucusless Diet. I watched him on videotape lecturing at his School of Natural Healing. He founded the school in 1953.

In his youth, Dr. Christopher became interested in natural healing when he saw the positive results his mother achieved with naturopathic healing. His enthusiasm increased when he found he was able to cure himself of cancer using natural methods. Dr. Christopher went on to become a Naturopathic Doctor and is hailed as America's foremost herbalist.

What impressed me most about Dr. Christopher was his willingness to help people in need, even when doctors gave up on them. The following example of his commitment to help mankind will forever be pressed upon my heart.

During a severe snowstorm in Utah the mother of a very ill child called Dr. Christopher. She told him that their family doctor said there was nothing he could do for the child and he wouldn't travel to examine the baby during the snowstorm. He also said, if the weather cleared the next day he would be there in the morning to sign the death certificate.

Without any hesitation, Dr. Christopher drove fifty miles in freezing cold snowy weather to help this woman's baby. When he arrived, he saw that the baby had a severe case of pneumonia and immediately performed a hydrotherapy treatment. He left further instructions for the mother, before heading back out into the storm for the fifty-mile drive home.

The next morning, Dr. Christopher received a phone call from the baby's mother thanking him for saving her child's life.

In his video lectures, Dr. Christopher explained how simple it is to keep the body healthy when given the proper cleansing and nourishment.

He emphasized the "Mucusless Diet" and the importance of this diet during illness and disease. Dr. Christopher continued to share that the purpose of the Mucusless Diet is to eliminate mucus from the body. With the mucus out, natural healing is easier to obtain.

This made perfect sense to me. From that moment forward I knew I was going to continue on with the Mucusless Diet. A clear confirmation that I was on the right healing path came to me after learning that Dr. Schulze was Dr. Christopher's student, at the School of Natural Healing.

Dr. Christopher believed that in order to heal the body completely, all mucus-forming foods must be eliminated from the diet. There was no need to put mucus into the body faster than it could be eliminated. By eliminating mucus from the body... the sinuses, the bronchi, and the lungs are cleared and best of all... constipating mucus in the tissues of the body, from the head to the bottom of the feet, are cleared.

The Foundation of the Mucusless Diet I Followed for the First Year of my Healing:

I AVOIDED: All meat, anything with white flour in it, processed sugar, and all dairy. This may sound extreme but it isn't. It is much easier to eliminated these foods when you know how to prepare recipes without it.

The Lidle Café Cookbook in the back of this book is a great start.

The following denaturalized and inorganic food substances are harmful, mucus-forming and I eliminated them from my diet.

Salt. I substituted *sea salt*, coarsely ground organic pepper, powdered kelp and herbs. Black pepper is a nutritional herb and helps rebuild the body when used in its natural state.

When pepper is cooked, at high heat, it becomes an inorganic irritant.

Eggs. No eggs in any form.

Sugar. All sugar and sugar products that are refined and processed. Raw honey and blackstrap or sorghum molasses is O.K.

Meat. All red meat. A little bit of fish or free range chicken which has not been contaminated by chemicals, inoculated with formaldehyde or any other preserving substances is O.K. *I chose not to eat any meat for the year.* It's not that difficult. After a few weeks of being off meat I lost the craving.

Milk. I eliminated all dairy and dairy products including: butter, cheese, cottage cheese (cheese is one of the most constipating foods. Even today, the few times I do eat cheese I immediately get constipated and can't go without an herbal aid), sour cream, whipped cream, ice cream, yogurt, milk, etc. All milk products are mucus forming. I've battled with eczema most of my life. Since eliminating dairy from my diet, I don't have a speck of eczema.

Flour. White Flour when heated and baked at high temperatures, changes to a mucus-forming substance. All of my allergies disappeared when I stopped eating white flour products.

After eliminating all of the above foods from my diet, symptoms of Tourette's syndrome almost all disappeared. I had my attention back and I felt so clear and present.

➤ Read what the *Alternative Medicine Digest*, Issue 15 has to say about mucus:

"A material similar to paper-mache can develop in the lining of the small and large intestines as a result of eating white flour products combined with fluid and cellulose, which is found in vegetables. When you eat other foods that produce mucus such as dairy and sugar products, the result is a rubbery-like material that combines with the paper-mache lining, and it builds up even faster.

As this sticky **mucoid** false lining builds up in the small intestines, it **blocks absorption of essential nutrients** into the blood stream and produces a hiding place in both intestines for bacteria, fungi, yeast and parasites that are harmful to human health.

When these abnormal life forms start growing too freely in the intestines, they kill off L. Acidophilus and other "friendly" bacteria. They also create a situation called dysbiosis (an imbalance among intestinal microflora) in which the contents of the intestines putrefy and harmful chemicals are generated.

The result is a toxic bowel and a body-wide condition of toxicity as toxins leech out of the intestines into other tissue."

———————————————

My Healing Diet the First Year

* My diet consisted of **75% *uncooked, raw foods***
  including: All vegetables, all fruits, raw pre-
  soaked nuts and seeds and lots of fresh juiced
  vegetables with carrots always as the base.

* ***25% of my diet was cooked.*** The only cooked
  foods I ate were: Veggie sandwiches with
  Ezekiel bread, potatoes, brown rice, hummus,
  steamed veggies, lots of nutritional vegetable broth,
  vegetable soup, black beans and vegetarian chili
  *(I did eat everything on Thanksgiving, I couldn't
  resist, it was delicious.)*

* Once or twice **each day, I drank a green super
  nutrition drink.** Many days I drank 1 oz of wheat
  grass juice. (If you have questions about what
  ingredients to look for in a green nutritional drink call
  me or email me at: 480-948-3386 or ablhealth@aol.com

* I put three tablespoons of either flaxseed oil or fresh
  ground flaxseeds in juice, at least five days a week.

* Each month I took at least two ounces of
  Echinacea and drank a lot of Red Clover Tea.

* From the fourth month on, *for eight months,* I took
  Native American Black Salve internally every day.

Three-day " Apple Juice" Cleanse

Dr. Christopher believed the purpose of this cleansing program is to purify the body so healing can result.

I did the three-day juice cleanse toward the end of my first year of healing.

The three-day juice cleanse consists of drinking prune juice first thing in the morning, drinking juice and water throughout the day, and taking olive oil three times a day. The cleansing juices recommended are: carrot, apple, grape or citrus. If you're going to use bottle juices, make sure there is no added sugar.

After doing several of these cleanses the best results I received were from *freshly juiced granny smith apples*. Bottled apple juice and grape juice bloated me and gave me cramps.

Keep in mind that we are unique and our bodies are different. What works for one person may not work for another, so experiment with different juices and discover which works best for you.

I found it was best to begin eating mostly raw foods, one week prior to the juice cleanse.

Into my second and third year, when I didn't prepare ahead of time, I experienced withdrawal symptoms that included headaches and dizziness. When this happened, I ate a piece of apple and it helped.

After completing the three-day cleanse, I continued to drink fresh juices, raw or lightly steamed vegetables and fruits for four to five days.

I may have developed intestinal and digestive problems if I ate irritating and mucus forming foods immediately after the cleanse so, I WAS CAREFULL.

Important: *Please consult your physician or a qualified health practitioner before doing this cleanse, especially if you have blood sugar issues or high blood pressure.*

A Sample Schedule of the
Three-day Apple Juice Cleanse, I follow:

7:00	16oz of Prune Juice and 1-2 tbs. of Cold Pressed Virgin Olive Oil
7:30	8oz of Distilled Water
8:00	8oz of Fresh Apple Juice with one tbs. of Olive Oil
8:30	8oz of Distilled Water

Alternate water and juice each half-hour until 12:00 noon

12:00	8oz of Fresh Apple Juice and one tbs. of Olive Oil
12:30	8oz of Distilled Water
1:00	8oz of Fresh Apple Juice

I continued this same sequence, alternating water and juice each half-hour until 6:00 p.m.

6:00	8oz of Fresh Apple Juice with one tbs. of Olive Oil
6:30	8oz of Distilled Water
7:00	8oz of Fresh Apple Juice

After 7:30, I drink only water until bedtime or if I feel a little lightheaded I eat an apple (sometimes I stopped by 5:00)
*this schedule is the same for all three days

Chapter Eight

Native American Black Salve

Four months into my healing program I was introduced to Native American Black Salve.

Before I give you the details of my personal positive
experience with the salve you should know its history. The
salve has been available for over 100 years. An early
pioneer family was introduced to the salve by Native
American Indians. The formula was passed down in that
family for three generations. For many years the salve has
been used to eliminate cancer not only in humans but also in
cows, to save herds of calves from early viral diseases,
sarcoids on horses, and abnormal tissue growths in all kinds
of animals.

One of the original family members that made the
salve was the first to use it internally. He had been
diagnosed with colon cancer in the 1960's. After he checked

himself in to the hospital for surgery, the night before, he took the first dose of black salve in a capsule without telling his doctors.

The next morning they postponed his surgery because he was having cramps, as the salve had started to work in his system. He then continued to take the salve for five more days. On the fifth day he said he passed a large quantity of black vile smelling feces, apparently the growth itself. When the doctors took x-rays, they discovered the cancerous growth was gone. He lived another twenty-five years, without colon cancer returning.

A woman who eliminated cancer from her breast using the black salve telephoned me. She said she was told that I was healing myself using natural methods. After a lengthy conversation, we enthusiastically set a time to meet.

She came to my home and shared her healing testimony in detail. She was diagnosed with breast cancer and a needle biopsy revealed the cancer was very advanced. A friend told her about the black salve, and so she gave it a shot. After three months of taking it internally, she went back for another biopsy and the cancer was gone. Her healing was not without pain.

After the first month, her breast became excruciatingly sore at times. It turned black and blue (where the cancer was) and she was afraid it was going to come through her skin. It never did. She also chose to not undergo any conventional treatment.

What I was hearing sounded terrific, but at that time my course of healing was already planned out and I didn't want to deviate.

If you have cancer or any other disease and are following a natural healing path – either totally or in conjunction with conventional treatment, you'll agree that everyone has something else you should be taking or trying.

You begin doubting yourself and wonder, "What more should I be taking?" It's too overwhelming because there are so many things that are good for you and do work. After months of ingesting many herbal formulas, I decided to take the maximum of FIVE, cancer fighting and immune building supplements. I wanted to simplify my healing plan.

For some reason, I couldn't stop thinking about the black salve. Through the natural healing grapevine, I heard more and more about this salve. So, I called this woman back and asked if I could get some. Within a few days I began taking it internally, once a day.

On the fifth day of taking the salve I got really ill from it. I took it with mashed potatoes and lots of raw garlic. They didn't mix. Honestly, I was a little worried. After a few hours I had the urgency to go to the bathroom. It was amazing how much reddish-brown diarrhea came out of me. As you already know, I was thoroughly cleansed at this point. Where was this coming from?

I remember thinking, "This looks like my hair dye." I felt a little better at that point. Within an hour, I felt a mild electrical type of a shock or vibration in my left breast and within a minute, three in my right breast. This didn't alarm me because I remembered the woman's testimony of it being painful for her. That evening the same vibrating electrical shock happened under my ribs on the left side. In the middle of the night, I was woken up by severe pain behind my right knee.

My immediate thoughts were that the salve got the rest of the cancer in my left breast and in my right breast (I probably had cancer in my right breast as well). Years ago, I had a lump develop under my left rib and I thought I strained something playing tennis. It soon went away. During high school, I had knee surgery on my right knee. Scar tissue developed and I believe the salve cleaned up the scar tissue. I heard the salve has the ability to do that. The next day, my stomach was still tender so I stopped taking the salve for a few days.

For the next eight months,
I continued taking the black salve,
and continue to take today for
four months every year.

During the sixth month into my healing program, my nipple returned to completely normal. The puckering was gone and my nipple worked again. I really believe I was healed at this point.

BEWARE: *Not all salves are the same. If the salve is sold without instructions... I would NOT purchase it. I spoke with someone who had personal experience with the salve. If directions are not followed accurately results may vary and be dangerous. Consult a naturopathic physician.*

- Chapter Nine -

What I Do To Keep My Healing

Skin Brushing

Paavo O. Airola, ND, Ph.D. writes, "The number one cause of all so-called degenerative diseases and premature aging is to be found in the derangement of cell metabolism and in slowed-down cell regeneration. This derangement is mainly caused by the accumulation of waste products in the tissues which interferes with the nourishment and oxygenation of the cells."

During the first three months of my healing program, I brushed my entire body everyday. Our largest eliminative organ is our skin, which is made up of hundreds of thousands of sweat glands. It's estimated that one-third of the body's impurities are released through the skin. One pound of waste products are eliminating through our skin daily.

When we don't keep the pores open they become clogged. The impurities are trapped and reabsorbed into the body and released into tissues. In Dr. Airola's book, I've also read that the chemical analysis of sweat shows it to have uric acid, which is the same waste product and normal component of urine.

Benefits of skin brushing:

- The dead layers of skin and impurities are removed.
- It stimulates the blood circulation in the underlying tissue and organ.
- It has a rejuvenating effect on the nervous system by stimulating the nerve endings in the skin. It contributes to healthier muscle tone and a better distribution of fat deposits. You'll feel better all around, because you're becoming proactive in your health program.

Start skin brushing, here's how you do it:

✓ First, be sure to use a natural bristle brush, then before you shower begin by brushing the bottoms of your feet.

✓ Proceed to your legs and then brush the rest of the body. It's very important to brush upward or downward toward your HEART. After using the skin brush a few times wash it with soap and let it dry in the sunlight.

The Importance of Exercise

"Use it or lose it." The fluid in the lymphatic system, which houses the immune cells, depends largely on exercise to be circulated. Twenty to thirty minutes of exercise a day is deemed sufficient to insure proper circulation.

Exercise also builds the heart and enables it to pump blood throughout the entire body. If you're not exercising regularly because of weather or for any other reason, try a mini-bouncer (looks like a mini trampoline) and bounce on it every day for at least 20 minutes. *Exercise makes you feel good, once you get past the procrastination of doing it!*

Deep Breathing

Air is the breath of life. Deep breathing enhances the supply of oxygen to every cell in the body and also aids in cleansing the bloodstream.

➢ Simply take a few minutes, three or four times a day. Breathe through your nose, hold it as long as you can, then exhale slowly through your mouth.

➢ Deep breathing is also effective to do when you feel stressed or anxious. It will calm you down, instantly.

A person can survive 110 days without food, 12 days without water, but only a few minutes without oxygen.

Sunshine

Sunlight is necessary for the synthesis of vitamin D. The ultraviolet rays act on the cholesterol substances contained in the skin to form a chemical called cholecalciferol, also known as vitamin D-3. This Vitamin D is an important vitamin because it regulates the calcium and phosphorus metabolism of the body.

Studies have shown the best time to get these rays without harmful effects are before 10:00 o'clock in the morning and after 4:00 o'clock in the afternoon.

Flaxseeds

Flaxseeds are one of my favorite morning additions to breakfast. Most mornings I add two to three tablespoons of ground flaxseed to juice or in cereal. The mornings I have only a super nutrition drink, I add some flaxseed oil.

Flaxseed is a rich source of the omega 3 fatty acid, alpha-linolenic acid. This fatty acid is considered essential, meaning your body cannot make it, but requires it and so must derive all of it from the diet. Our American diet is sorely lacking in this healing fat.

Omega 3 fatty acids are necessary for proper infant growth and development. They are especially important in the formation of a healthy nervous system and to help keep that nervous system functioning properly. It has been shown to be useful in the treatment of multiple sclerosis, and behavioral problems like ADD, depression and bipolar disorder in adults and children. *(For me, it certainly seems to help symptoms associated with Tourette syndrome).*

Omega 3 fats are also important in modifying the body's inflammatory response, making them very helpful in the treatment of inflammatory diseases like allergies, asthma, arthritis and eczema. Studies have shown that omega 3 fats can lower blood pressure, and can lower blood cholesterol and triglycerides. The most exciting health benefit from flax is its impact on the number one killer in our country, heart disease.

Vitamin C

Vitamin C is the champion of vitamins, the artillery so to speak. It is recognized that Vitamin C in the body inhibits cancer growth. It has been observed to inhibit cancer from spreading within the body by neutralizing a particular enzyme, produced by the cancer cell, which would otherwise aid the cancer in spreading.

Vitamin C is also a powerful antioxidant and stimulates the immune system to attack abnormal cells. Dr. Paavo Airola in his book, 'How To Get Well', concludes that a person needs 100mg. to 200 mg. of vitamin C a day for maintenance of normal, healthy functions of the body. However, when a person takes vitamin C in huge doses, 5,000 to 10,000 mg. a day, it will assume a totally different function and can perform miracles such as:

✓ Killing pathogenic bacteria and acting as an antibiotic.
✓ Preventing and curing colds and infections, having a natural antihistamine activity.
✓ Being a potent antitoxin.
✓ Speeding the healing process.
✓ Preventing premature aging by strengthening the collagen and preventing the degenerative process.

Garlic

Throughout this book I reference Dr. Paavo Airola because I respect his knowledge and his dedication as a leading authority on biological medicine. Dr. Airola described garlic as, "A much neglected wonder food with amazing nutritional and medical properties, and the King of the vegetable kingdom."

His research of the world's scientific literature confirms the following facts: Garlic has been proven to be effective in treating allergies, arthritis, arteriosclerosis, cancer, diabetes, hypoglycemia, fungus disease, candidiasis, gastrointestinal disorders, colitis, asthma, bronchitis and pneumonia.

Research indicates the trace minerals germanium and selenium, both concentrated in garlic, are important in proper immune function.

It's a good thing my husband loves garlic as much as I do. We consume at least 3-5 bulbs of garlic a week.

Chiropractic

Practitioners of chiropractic therapy believe that dysfunction of one part of the body often affects the function of other, not necessarily connected, parts.

Health is restored by manipulating bones, soft tissues, or by realigning body parts. Disease prevention and health promotion through proper diet, exercise and lifestyle are other important features of chiropractic medicine. My experience with chiropractic care has been very positive.

In Addition:

- ➤ I take a powerful immune support which includes: Echinacea, Pau D'Arco, Garlic, Cats Claw, Cayenne, Usnea Lichen, Maitake and Shitake mushroom.

- ➤ Three to four times a week I add cayenne pepper to water and drink it.

- ➤ I take a female herbal balance formula which contains: Wild Yam, Black Cohosh, Chaste Tree, Angelica, Licorice, Lobelia, Ginger, Skullcap, Horsetail Herb, Hops and Damiana.

- ➤ Once or twice a week I have a tablespoon of blackstrap molasses in a little bit of water.

- ➤ Deep breathing exercises a few times a day.

- ➤ Steam sauna with aromatherapy a few times a week.

- ➤ Exercise every other day for at least one hour.

- ➤ I live in the moment and not worry too much about the future.

- ➤ I laugh a lot! and play a lot! We take life so seriously that we forget how to enjoy it.

How Do I Know I'm Free of Cancer?

Not too long ago, I had a series of blood tests run.
The name of the tests were a CHEMPANEL, BASIC,
CBC W/DIFF/PLT

My White Blood Count was 8.9. The normal range is
4.0-11.0. I was really happy about that.

My calcium was 10. The normal range is 8.4 –10.2.

My Alkaline Phospatase was 75 and the normal is 39-117
(the naturopathic doctor who ordered these tests said this
test would indicate if cancer was in my bones). I was in the
normal range.

The CA 27.29 is a test approved by the Food and Drug
Administration for monitoring breast cancer patients with
metastatic disease and as an adjunct to established
techniques for detecting recurrence in patients previously
treated for stage II or stage III breast cancer. (I was very
happy about this result).

As far as being free from cancer? I'm not in fear of it ever
taking over my body so in this respect, I'm free from cancer.
Cancer doesn't scare me. These past four and a half years
have given me powerful ammunition to fight it. So, if it
does come back, my immune system will defeat it. This is
why it is so important to keep the immune system strong
and alert.

Chapter Ten

Getting a "Fresh Start"

Most people don't realize how easy it is to transition into a healthier lifestyle. Unfortunately they've never been exposed to it.

Many also think healthier foods are much more expensive so they don't venture out to buy them. Unfortunately, some are more expensive while others are not. I'm beginning to keep track of the cost of the ingredients and I find that it's not that much more and surprisingly sometimes less!

I shop at natural food markets and at farmers markets.

The salad dressings I make from scratch are inexpensive and they don't have added chemicals. In the Fresh Start Shopping Guide, I also list a few salad dressings in a bottle that are delicious and not expensive.

The biggest objection I hear from parents is, " I can't get my kids to eat healthy foods." Yes, there are a lot of packaged health foods that are terrible... and there are a lot of good ones. You need to try a variety of foods. I agree that most cheese made from soy tastes like cardboard so....I MAKE MY OWN... and it only takes 10-15 minutes.

I can empathize with parents... but... come on... who's in charge... the kids or the parents? When a child gets hungry enough they will eat the healthier foods presented to them (especially if they are colorful and fun to eat).

At one of the Fresh Start cooking classes I teach, a young mother attended. She was so surprised at how good the desserts we made were. The next morning she gave her young son a taste of the Energy Candy and he loved them... so much... he ate six of them.

That same day she called me and said, *"The day he ate the Energy Candy was one of the first days, she can remember, he didn't have refined sugar."* The recipe for the Energy Candy is in the recipe section.

As I'm writing this chapter I'm wondering how can I best give you an example of the variety of healthy foods you and your family can eat. The following guide is what I came up with. These are some of the foods we eat in our home.

"The greatest discovery
a person can make
is to realize
that they can change
their life
by changing their
attitude"

"Fresh Start" Choices
Breakfast, Lunch & Dinner

It's easy to eat healthier meals if you know what to buy and how to prepare them. The following suggestions are foods we eat in our household. It's very important to have healthy foods in your kitchen at all times. When you do it's easier to eat at home and not run out for fast food.

Bill and I spend about $75 a week for groceries. This is when we eat at home and not at restaurants.

Breakfast:

* My husband and I always begin each day with a glass of purified water, sometimes warm with the juice of 1 lemon.

* Nutritional Green Breakfast Drink mixed with juice, fruit and ground flaxseeds or flaxseed oil

* Whole grain cereal with raisins, bananas, flaxseeds, almond or rice milk

* Whole grain or sprouted whole grain toast with raw almond butter and fruit sweetened jam

* Bowl of a variety of fresh fruit: cantaloupe, banana, peaches, pears, apples (whatever is in season) and a whole grain muffin sweetened with honey not refined sugar

* Fruit smoothie or fresh orange juice and a piece of whole grain toast with raw almond butter

* Scrambled tofu with fresh fruit

* Breakfast wraps (organic eggs or tofu with sautéed tomatoes, onions, peppers, zucchini, and or corn)

* Fresh squeezed carrot, apple and ginger juice

* Tortilla Española (fabulous for brunch!)

* Sliced bananas with raw carob powder sprinkled on top

* Juice and Energy Candy *(uncooked, no refined sugar)*

* Juice and No-Bake Apple Pie

* Juice and Orange, Date Squares

* Whole grain or Rice Waffles *(uncooked, no refined sugar)*

* Buckwheat, Oat Flour and Flaxseed Pancakes

Lunch and/or Dinner

* Fresh Creamy Corn Chowder

* Vegetarian Chili

* Potato, Celery & Leek Soup

* Refreshing Carrot Soup

* Fresh vegetable juice (I always have carrot as my base) and celery, parsley, apples, ginger, beet, or spinach

* Garden Salad Wrap

*Roasted Eggplant, Corn & Zucchini Wrap

*Garden Burger with Potato Salad with Almonnaise

*Raw Nut Butter and Jam Sandwich

*Vegetable Paté Sandwich

*Medley Crunch Salad with Toasted Spinach or Whole Wheat Tortilla

*Hummus Dip with Fresh Vegetables

*Marinara Sauce with Angel Hair Zucchini, Sweet Potato or Squash

*Creamy Vegetables and Brown Rice

*The Lidle Café Potato Casserole Surprise

*Spicy Green Beans & Mashed Potatoes

*Corn Tacos with sautéed onions, green peppers, black beans, brown rice and salsa

*Pistachio Pesto Pasta

*Fruit Fondue

*Zesty lemon Pudding

*No-Bake Apple Pie (no refined sugar)

*Orange, Date Bars (uncooked with no refined sugar)

*Energy Candy

*A few times each month, my husband likes to have a piece of organic free range chicken, turkey or deep sea fish. It's seems we have less and less fish as time goes on.

One secret to feeling better and eating less is to
STOP nibbling between meals.
This gives the body a chance to digest
breakfast, lunch and dinner.

Where Do I Get My Protein?

"Where do you get your protein?", is one of the most frequent questions I get asked. The only meat I've had in over four years is a little turkey at Thanksgiving, a little deep sea once in a while.

Even without eating lots of meat, I STILL HAVE MUSCLE. I haven't withered away. This proves to me that I don't need meat in my diet. I get protein from vegetables, raw nuts and seeds, organic tofu and flaxseed. I build my blood with blackstrap molasses and lots of blueberries, raspberries, grape and blueberry juice. My husband on the other hand, after four years of eating the same way I do, is adding a little more organic free-range turkey to his diet. He says he feels better.

Dr. N.W. Walker in his book "Become Younger" explains the protein question the best. Here's what he says:

The human body cannot utilize a complete protein, such as the meat of animals, fish or birds as a complete product.

"The human body must break it down and disintegrate it into the atoms and molecules composing it. It then recombines such atoms as are necessary to build up the particular amino acids required at the moment, which may be entirely different from those in the meat we eat.

During this process of breaking down and disintegrating, the digestive system is really working overtime, which results in the generation of excessive quantities of uric acid.

This acid gets into muscles. Sooner or later the saturation point is reached in some of the muscles and the acid crystallizes, forming tiny uric acid crystal in the shape of microscopic hard, sharp splinters. It is then that the real trouble begins, because the movement of these muscles cases these tiny sharp points to pierce the sheathing of the nerves and the *resulting torture is labeled rheumatism, neuritis or sciatica, etc.*"

Do you ever notice how tired people are after eating a holiday meal filled with meat and starches? How they want to go to take a nap and go to sleep. If these foods are so good for us, why do they make us tired instead of giving us energy? Notice how after eating a meal full of vegetables and fresh fruit and juices you feel energized? Well, "The proof is in the pudding," so to speak.

I don't believe eating meat once in a while is so harmful. I do believe the unnatural feeding of animals and the inhumane processing of their meat is disgusting! I read somewhere recently, that animals know when they are going to be slaughtered. The adrenaline produced at this time is an enormous amount. This adrenaline is stored in their meat and is still present at the time we cook and eat it. Don't people and kids seem more quick to lose their tempers now a days?

Why I Prefer *Not* To Eat Dairy Products

First of all, each time I do, I begin to rash and eczema breaks out on my ears and my forearms.

Dr. N. W. Walker explains why dairy is unnecessary for human consumption. He says, "Milk is intended by Nature to grow the bone structure of the particular animal from which it comes. Cow's milk contains 300% more casein than does mother's milk, and is intended to grow the calf to maturity of about three quarters of a ton.

The vast percentage of casein in cow's milk, however, is not digested and assimilated in the human body. Except in rare instances, milk is useless as a human food as it clogs up the system with mucus. This mucus lodges usually in the sinus cavities, in the breathing channels and in many other vital parts of the system."

Do you notice how young girls are developing breasts at a younger age and beginning their menstrual cycles at an earlier age? Investigate these statements and learn what organization created the food chart for our schools to follow. You may be very surprised.

"Fresh Start" Shopping List

The following list will help you to get started adding healthier foods into your daily life. *If your local grocery or health food store does not stock these items ask them to order them for you.*

If they won't, then you may be able to get these items in quantity from Mountain People Distributing. There is a minimum dollar requirement. Ask a few of your friends to choose the foods they want and do a collective co-op order. I believe they can deliver to most states. 800-679-6733

SPICES: I keep these spices stocked at all times.

The Spice Hunter: name brand
All Purpose Chef's Shake
Pesto Seasoning
Coriander
Fajita Seasoning
Italian Seasoning (organic)

Frontier: name brand
Oregano Leaf (organic)

A. Vogel: name brand
Herbamare organic herb seasoning salt

Roasted Minced Garlic
Celtic Sea Salt
Bill's Best Chik'Nish Seasoning
Hungarian Hot Paprika
Organic Vegetarian Worcestershire Sauce

PASTA
Lunderg and Ancient Quinoa Harvest: name brands
-Organic Soy Pasta
-Brown Rice Pasta
-Spelt Pasta
-Lentil Pasta
-Quinoa Pasta *(pronounced Keen-wa)*

FROZEN FOODS
Amy's Brand Name is always good:
Organic pizza, Enchiladas & more

BREAD & TORTILLAS & TACO SHELSS
-Ezekiel Bread
-Spelt and Sprouted Grain Breads
-Sprouted Whole Wheat or Whole Wheat
  (look for tortillas without chemicals)
-Bearitos – Organic Corn Taco Shells

BEANS & RICE
-Black Beans
-Navy Beans
-Pinto Beans
-Brown Rice
-Barley

RAW ALMOND BUTTER & JAMS
Without processed sugar or high fructose syrup or
corn syrup

FROZEN WAFFLES
Van's Wheat Free Waffles

VEGETABLES

It's easier for you to eat healthy if you have as many of these veggies in your refrigerator at all times. If you buy organic they don't last as long but they taste better and are better for you.

- ➢ Carrots
- ➢ Celery
- ➢ Potatoes
- ➢ Garlic
- ➢ Tomatoes
- ➢ Red, Green & Yellow Bell Pepper
- ➢ Cucumber
- ➢ Corn
- ➢ Eggplant
- ➢ Zucchini
- ➢ Broccoli
- ➢ Cauliflower
- ➢ Long Green Beans
- ➢ Onions & Shallots
- ➢ Parsley

NUTS & SEEDS

-Raw Almonds
-Cashews
-Walnuts
-Pumpkin Seeds
-Sesame Seeds
-Sunflower Seeds

*Soaking nuts and seeds in water for 8 hours before eating starts the enzyme action. After soaking, pat dry with paper towel and always refrigerate after...only lasts three days.

FROZEN FRUIT
Blueberries, Raspberries, Mango, Strawberries
Is great in cereal, fruit smoothies and eat it alone... berries are good for the blood.

BOXED CEREAL
-Health Valley Organic Fiber 7 Multigrain Flakes
-Arrowhead Mills Organic Amaranth Flakes
-Erewhon Crispy Brown Rice (just like Rice Krispies)

GOLDEN FLAXSEED
Grind and put on cereal or in juice

HUMMUS DIP
Garbanzo Beans, garlic, lemon and sea salt
This is always a good dip for corn chips, to spread on sandwiches and to dip veggies in. Try mixing salsa in with the hummus. It's great! Look for it in the refrigerated section.)

EXTRA VIRGIN OLIVE OIL

BLUE CORN TORTILLA CHIPS

SALAD DRESSING
Annies Naturals – brand name
-Caesar
-Tuscany Dressing

I prefer to make it fresh, but when I don't have time these bottled dressings are good..

RAISIN BRAN MUFFINS from FOOD FOR LIFE

Reading Labels

What if someone were to tell you that a chemical added to food could cause brain damage in you and your children, future learning and emotional difficulties?

Suppose evidence was presented to you strongly suggesting that the artificial sweetener in your diet soft drink may cause brain tumors, and that the number of brain tumors reported since the introduction of this artificial sweetener has risen dramatically?

There is growing evidence that 'Excitotoxins" play a significant role in a wide range of degenerative brain diseases in adults.   Diseases like Parkinson's disease, Alzheimer's disease, Huntington's disease, Amyotrophic Lateral Sclerosis and more disorder of the nervous system. "Excitotoxin" accumulation in the brain is being linked to other disorders such as strokes, seizures, migraine headaches and even AIDS dementia.

What if you learned that the food industry
disguises many of these "Excitotoxin additives",
so they will not be recognized?

What are "Excitotoxins, how do they work?

They are chemical compounds. When neurons are exposed to these substances, they become very excited and fire impulses rapidly until they reach a state of extreme exhaustion. Hours later, these neurons suddenly die, as if they were excited to death. This is why neuro-scientists labeled these chemicals, "Excitotoxins".

Why are they added to food? They stimulate the taste cells in the tongue and greatly enhance the taste of the foods they are added to. *They are often used in soups, sauces, gravy mixes, low fat foods and frozen diet foods.*

For thousands of years, Japanese cooks added an ingredient (made from sea weed) to their foods, to enhance the flavor. During the last century the active chemical in this taste-enhancing ingredient was isolated. *This chemical is called MSG, monosodium glutamate.*

After World War II, American food manufacturers were adding millions of pounds of MSG to processed foods each year. MSG was thought to be completely safe and many cookbooks even recommended adding MSG to their recipes. The amount of MSG added to foods has doubled every decade since the 1940's. In 1957, two ophthalmologists, Lucas and Newhouse, tested MSG on infant mice to study eye disease. *When they examined the eye tissues of the mice, they discovered the MSG had destroyed all of the nerve cells in the inner layers of the retina, which are the visual receptor cells of the eye.*

*Even after this alarming discovery MSG
continued to be added to foods.*

Approximately ten years later, John W. Olney, MD, a neuroscientist repeated Lucas' and Newhouses's experiment in infant mice. He found that not only was the MSG toxic to the retina, it was also toxic to the brain.

He discovered that specialized cells in a critical area of the mice's brain, the hypothalamus, were destroyed after a single dose of MSG.

One might think these alarming findings would have put a ban on MSG being added to foods, especially BABY FOODS. Food manufacturers continued to add MSG and hydrolyzed vegetable protein (a compound containing three 'Excitotoxin" additives and some MSG) to a variety of foods, including baby foods.

The concentrations of MSG found in baby foods was equal to that used to create brain lesions in experimental animals. Tests showed immature animals (babies) were found to be MORE vulnerable to the toxic effects of MSG than were older animals (adults).

Dr. Olney gave his testimony before a congressional committee and the food manufacturers agreed to remove MSG from baby foods. OR DID THEY?

Instead of adding pure MSG, they added hydrolyzed vegetable protein. This continued for seven years and even today there is evidence that "Excitotoxins" are added to baby foods.

Hydrolyzed vegetable protein, also referred to as vegetable protein or plant protein is said to be a safe natural substance made from plants. Yes, it is made from vegetables. *Vegetables unfit for sale to consumers. They are selected for their high content of glutamate.

The extraction process of hydrolysis involves boiling these vegetables in a vat of acid and then neutralizing them with caustic soda. A brown sludge that collects on top is then scraped off and allowed to dry. The end result is a brown powder high in three known "Excitotoxins": glutamate, aspartate, and cystoic acid, which convert in the body to cysteine.

These "Excitotoxins" are then added directly to foods, or mixed with other ingredients and added to foods to enhance their flavor.

Yuk! Yuk! Yuk!

Some neuroscientsists believe that exposure to these powerful compounds early in life could cause developmental brain defects producing learning difficulties and behavioral problems, as the child grows older. Violent behavior may also be a result.

As it stands today, the word monosodium glutamate (MSG) is not required on food labels unless the product contains 100% pure MSG.

For example, if broth is used to make soup, and the broth contains pure MSG, MSG does not have to be listed as an ingredient... but if the broth is sold alone, it must appear on the label.

The source for the above information was gathered from the book entitled, "Excitotoxins, The Taste That Kills" authored by Russell L. Blaylock, MD. I highly recommend this book for all those seeking better health. A few years ago I met Dr. Blaylock and can attest to his fine character. *Investigate this issue further for yourself.*

Hidden Sources of MSG

Monosodium Glutamate
Hydrolyzed Vegetable Protein
Hydrolyzed Protein
Hydrolyzed Plan Protein
Plant Protein Extract
Autolyzed Yeast
Hydrolyzed Oat Flour
Sodium Caseinate
Calcium Caseinate
Yeast Extract
Textured Protein

Additives that frequently contain MSG

Malt Extract
Bouillon
Stock Flavoring
Natural Beef
Seasoning
Malt Flavoring
Broth
Natural Flavoring
Chicken Flavoring
Spices

*Don't panic or get overly alarmed.

*Do, take control and choose wisely the next time you go shopping.

*If you can, go through all of your foods at home and read the labels.

*It's not necessary to make a drastic lifestyle change, unless you are fighting a disease.

*Each step taken, leads closer to the goal of Better Health.

- Chapter Eleven -

Life Enhancing...
Important Health Principles

By having a basic knowledge of these health principles, it was easier for me to understand what my body was going through during the many cleansing and health building programs I experienced.

The few times I felt like quitting, I picked up a book and read about these principles. After I did, I was re-energized to get rid of the poisons in my body so it could heal itself.

You may already be familiar with these principles. If you are, I'm certain you'll agree to the important roles they play in natural healing.

If you're not familiar with these principles, the following summary will help you to understand the programs and understand why they worked as well as they did for me. For greater details on any topic of this overview, please refer to the books, listed in the bibliography.

➤ Internal Cleansing & Detoxification

Our bodies are in a continuous mode of detoxification every day. In much the same way our hearts beat and our lungs breathe. Our metabolic processes continuously encounter and dispose of a variety of toxins and poisons.

Some are cellular waste material of our own making which are toxic by-products of metabolism. Others consist of environmental pollutants, pesticides and poisons ingested into our systems through the air we breathe, the foods we eat and the water we drink. The bowel, liver, kidney's, lungs, skin, lymphatic system and the spleen assist with the removal of these toxins.

What Causes Internal Toxicity?

Many things can cause toxicity. Some of these include: constipation (stagnation) somewhere in the body, faulty digestion caused by improper diet and mal-absorption problems, environmental pollution and toxins, as well as, chemical preservatives and pesticides in our foods. Believe it or not, stress can also cause internal toxicity.

When we are not eliminating properly, wastes may not be expelled for days, weeks, months and even years. Over time the bowel walls become encrusted with old built up fecal matter, causing toxins to build up in the colon. To illustrate this point, imagine this built up fecal matter to be handfuls of raw hamburger meat that has been left sitting in 98 degrees for a week.

Constipation in the colon interferes with vital nutrients being absorbed through the intestinal walls and channeled to where they are needed. In the midst of this build up... toxins, parasites, worms and harmful bacteria are having a picnic - feeding, breeding and reproducing. *Ponder this point... if these parasites and worms feed off of the toxic waste and build up in our bodies... doesn't it make sense that they have to eliminate inside our bodies, as well?*

It gets worse! If the toxicity level gets really high, the blood capillaries lining the intestinal walls absorb these toxins into the bloodstream, and eventually invade and pollute the organs and cells. The same organs created to dispose of these toxins. When this happens the whole body becomes toxic and disease begins to manifest. By now the body may be in a state of auto-intoxication or in simpler terms, in a state of "SELF POISONING."

Lindsey Duncan, C.N. founder of the Home Nutrition Clinic in Santa Monica says, "This auto-intoxication lowers our overall feeling of health and vitality. We start to blame other factors such as aging on why we experience a lack of energy, why we don't have that 'zip' in our walk or that 'sparkle' in our eyes. Age has nothing to do with this depletion of energy and degenerating health. Ninety-nine percent of the time these complaints can be alleviated through internal cleansing techniques."

If you eat three meals a day, you must eliminate three times. Many people are not aware of this and think eliminating once a day or less is normal. Think about this... if you eat three times a day and eliminate only once where are the other two meals?

Do I Need Internal Cleansing?

Does your toilet need cleaning? Every one can benefit from internal cleansing. What would happen if we put over 100,000 miles on our cars and never changed the oil, air filter or spark plugs? Wouldn't the car run badly and eventually break down?

Or what if garbage collectors were on strike for six months, the temperature was 98 degrees and we didn't have plastic garbage bags to put the garbage in? So we piled garbage on top of garbage inside a hot garage. How would the garage smell? How many flies and rodents would come to feast on this mess?

These analogies are examples of what happens in our own intestinal system when we get constipated and allow our elimination channels to get clogged up.

Dr. John R. Christopher, ND, a renowned herbalist and creator of the "Mucusless Diet", believed that the bottom line cause of all disease is constipation. Constipation, in this given context, being a blockage somewhere in the body which results in the organs not being allowed to perform their God given duties.

Symptoms of a blockage may include; constipation, gas, fatigue, weight gain, excessive mucus, arthritis, poor skin, poor memory, lower backache, depression, body odor, bad breath, etc.

Cleansing and Nourishing the Body

An important key to feeling good is to cleanse and nourish the body with proper nutrition.

Think of cleansing the intestines inside the body in the same way you would peel the skin off of an orange. The inside of the orange has been shielded from insects, birds, and the elements. In somewhat the same way, the mucus and toxic build-up in the intestines is the same kind of shield, but in this case, the shield is not a protective one, and instead it is A HARMFUL ONE... blocking important nutrients and slowly poisoning the body. Cleansing the intestine peels away this layer of mucus and toxins, thus allowing nourishment to get through to feed the body.

No cleansing and detoxification program is complete without proper nutrition. While cleansing stay away from low vitality foods, overcooked and processed foods with chemical preservatives, fried foods, soda (yes, even diet soda), refined products containing sugar, white flour products, salt (except sea salt), saturated fats, meat, caffeine, alcohol, and nicotine.

During a cleanse it is beneficial to give your digestive tract a well deserved break, so it can work on helping rid the body of old waste and toxins.

Eat foods that give the body life and vitality including: (preferably organic) fresh vegetables, fresh fruits, slow cooked whole grains and pre-soaked raw nuts and seeds. These foods contain the necessary enzymes to aid in digestion and assimilation of nutrients, as well as, the necessary fibers to expedite intestinal transit time of foods.

Colon Cleansing

Enemas and/or colonics are extremely *important* during a cleansing program. Both involve using purified water to irrigate and flush out harmful toxins and poisons, old encrusted fecal matter, mucus strings, parasites, candida and worms from the bowel *(Never would I have believed worms and parasites lived in me before my cleansing. They did! I've seen them be expelled with my own eyes).*

If these toxins are not flushed out and remain in the colon, they will get re-absorbed into the bloodstream and tissue, potentially poisoning the whole body.

Dr. Paavo Airola, ND, Ph.D., a leading authority on biological medicine, explains in his book entitled, 'How to Get Well', that "Your body will try to get them out through other eliminative organs particularly through the kidneys, which as a result, will often be overloaded and even damaged."

After an enema or a colonic, it is very important to re-establish friendly bacteria into the body (rectal and orally).

➢ The Use of Herbs and Fibers

Adding herbs and fibers to a cleansing program will help expedite the elimination of accumulated toxins and waste. Herbs are nature's cleansers and are a complete food source. Herbs are rich in vitamins, minerals, amino acids and enzymes. They help the body's inherent function to accelerate and stimulate the cleansing process.

They boost the re-growth of cells and tissues and work with the body's defense system to build resistance to disease.

Fibers provide roughage and bulk necessary to absorb toxins and sweep them out of the digestive tract and elimination channels.

➢ The Importance of Drinking Water

Our bodies are made up of approximately 80% water. Water is second only to oxygen in sustaining life. Water is necessary during a cleansing program to aid in flushing out the toxins and waste from the body. It also transports nutrients, vitamins, minerals, proteins and sugars for assimilation. The recommended amount of pure water during a cleansing program is: 8-10, 16 ounce glasses each day. It should be noted that continuing to drink this amount of water after your cleanse is also extremely beneficial.

➢ The Importance of a Strong Immune System

Picture your immune system being the front defensive line of a football team. The mission of this defensive line (your white blood cells) is to stop the other team from getting through and scoring points. If the defensive line, your immune system, is weak or injured the other team (harmful germs and disease) get through causing damage and scoring points.

How do you build up your defensive line? One very important way is by what you eat or don't eat. A lifestyle filled with fresh vegetables, fruits, whole grains, nuts and seeds will help to build the defense line, your immune system. In addition, eliminate sugar and alcohol from your diet as they both lower the immune system. Maybe the most important and sometimes overlooked immune system booster is a positive attitude toward your health and your life.

➢ Why Antioxidants are so Important

Antioxidants are compounds that protect cells in the body from damage induced by unstable oxygen molecules called free radicals.

Free radicals are the body's enemy. They are believed to be responsible for predisposing the body to many forms of cancer.

Some sources containing antioxidants include: dark green leafy vegetables, carrots, bok choy, organic soy, yellow and orange fruits, beta-carotene, spirulina, vitamin C and vitamin E.

➢ The Importance of Enzymes

Enzymes virtually control everything that goes on in the body. Eating, breathing, sleeping, thinking and even our emotions are based on enzyme reaction. Our immune functions, hormone production, tissue replacement, utilization of vitamins, and the battle against toxic substances rely on enzymes.

We are alive because enzymes make it possible. Without them, seeds wouldn't sprout and fruits wouldn't ripen.

Enzymes are a substance that facilitate and promote a chemical reaction, but the substance itself is not consumed by the reaction. They snap nutrients apart enabling them to be assimilated by the body (if the body is not constipated by mucus, toxins and waste).

Enzymes can be classified into three groups:

- ❖ metabolic enzymes - control most of the metabolic reactions (they are required to build nutrients into blood, bones, teeth, nerves, organs and tissues).
- ❖ digestive enzymes - digest food
- ❖ food enzymes - not produced in our bodies, but are contained in the foods we eat (live foods).

Enzymes are produced in our glands, such as the liver and the pancreas. However, these glands don't produce all that are needed. Live foods usually contain the enzymes within them for the digestion of that food. Enzymes in fruit convert starch into sugar. Enzymes in nuts and seeds digest fat.

According to Tonita d'Raye, author of "Food Enzymes For Vibrant Health and Increased Longevity", enzymes are the body's workforce. Enzymes are similar to a construction crew who uses various materials including concrete and lumber to build a building. Enzymes can also be thought of as the demolition team that clean up the debris. Tonita d'Raye writes, "Just as the construction crew uses various materials to build a house, the enzyme workforce builds, repairs and cleans up our bodies, utilizing nutrients extracted from the proteins, carbohydrates and fats we ingest." However, in the same way a house built without a foundation will not last for long, our body cannot utilize essential vitamins, minerals, trace elements and other nutrients without enzymes (our body's foundation).

When foods are cooked at temperatures higher than 118 degrees Fahrenheit, most of the enzymes are destroyed.

This is why it's very important to eat as much live food as you can. Include garlic, onions and sprouts along with fresh fruits and vegetables. Avoid table salt, which may be an indirect enzyme inhibitor. Drink freshly made vegetable juices and include fiber in your diet.

Early signs of enzyme deficiency are digestive complaints such as heartburn, gas, bloating and belching. More symptoms of a lack of enzymes include, stomach aches, diarrhea, constipation, chronic fatigue, yeast infections, headaches and nutritional deficiencies.

An important key to weight loss may be as simple as the activity of enzymes in the body. Dr. David Galton at Tufts University School of Medicine tested people weighing 230-240 pounds. He found that virtually all of them were lacking lipase enzymes in their fatty tissues. Lipase, found abundantly in raw foods, is a fat-splitting enzyme that aids the body in digestion, the storage and distribution of fat and the burning of fat for energy. Lipase activity breaks down and dissolves fat throughout the body. Source: Food Enzymes For Vibrant Health and Increased Longevity.

Enzymes are specific: *protease* digests proteins; *amylase* digests complex carbohydrates; *maltase* and *sucrase* digest complex and simple sugars; *lactase* digests milk solids; *lipase* digest fats and *cellulase* digest fiber.

Chapter Twelve

What is the Cause of Cancer?

"*Modern medicine attributes most cases of cancer to changes in DNA that reduce or eliminate the normal controls over cellular growth, maturation and programmed cell death.* These changes are more likely to occur in people with certain genetic backgrounds and in persons infected by chronic viruses (e.g., viral hepatitis may lead to liver cancer). The ultimate cause that may influence the risk of cancer, is often the exposure to carcinogenic chemicals (including those found in nature) and/or to radiation (including natural cosmic and earthly radiation). Coupled with a failure of the immune system to eliminate the cancer cells at an early stage in their multiplication.

In the field of traditional Chinese medicine, propensities and the impact of viruses and radiation could not be known. However, the *Chinese have understood that something from the environment, some kind of toxin, was a likely contributor to development of the disease.*

The experience of the Chinese doctors points to emotional contributions to the development of cancer. In particular, depression (as in repressed anger), anxiety (worry, fearfulness, and excess circular thinking) and grief (usually because of the death of a loved one) are thought to result in stagnation of circulation.

If this circulatory disturbance continues, there may be a local accumulation – eventually to become the tumor mass – at the weak point in the body. An underlying weakness in an organ or other body tissue is what allows the problem of stagnancy in circulation to eventually overcome normal patterns of cellular growth. Thus, a tumor, or some other type of excessive cellular activity, occurs. Source: Subhuti Dharmananda, Ph.D., Director, Institute for Traditional Medicine, Portland, Oregon.

After reading both of these approaches, digesting them and then reflecting on my life --- I can comfortably claim that cancer manifested inside my body due to genetic weaknesses, chronic viruses and the emotional trauma's I've lived through.

I believe my father's abuse of alcohol and his resentment and anger toward his mother and father weakened and constipated his liver. He passed on this genetic weakness to me. Also, contracting infectious Hepatitis during my teenage years further weakened my liver and immune functions. Ecoli in my kidney weakened my immune system as well. The death of my father, sister and brother sent my immune system on an extended vacation. To top it all off, the abuse I was subjecting my body to from overeating toxic foods was the final invitation for cancer to come on in!

Being a worrywart all of my life didn't help matters. I used to be the 'Queen' of damaging Circular Thinking. This means that I used to play damaging dialogue over and over in my mind. I think this in itself should be classified as a dis-ease! Through all of this chaos, I always knew I deserved to be happy and healthy during my lifetime, but how could I, if I was sabotaging my life instead.

All of the above factors led me to the conclusion that disease in the body is not manifested by one thing in particular. It's a combination of both physical and emotional constipation (stagnation somewhere in the body and in the emotions).

You already know from reading this book how I've changed my eating habits to eliminate the physical constipation from my life. I've also learned to recognize the warning signals when I engage in damaging emotional stuff.

I let bothersome things go quickly. When I feel things are becoming overwhelming (they still do sometimes), I give them up to God.

I received my healing because I was willing to receive it. I was also willing to do the work involved to get well. Holding steadfast to the end result, no matter who was against my methods of getting there.

Forgiving those who have hurt me in the past was crucial. Without doing so, I'm not sure I could keep my healing.

Chapter Thirteen

What My Friends Are Saying

Sharon, Linda and Michal will be sharing their thoughts with you. They are in this picture. It was taken in my back yard the day of my wedding.

From left to right: Sharon, Linda, Glady's (Bill's mother), me, Klara (my mother), Michal and Debbie.

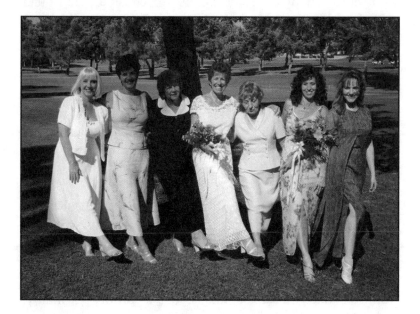

Michal

*My best friend, whom I think of as my sister. I've known
Michal for twenty-seven years!*

It was a typical July day in Israel, hot, sticky and
muggy. Like everyone, I was holed up in my apartment
trying to stay cool in the mid-afternoon heat, looking for
something entertaining to watch on television. I've gotten
used to screening my calls, but for some reason decided to
pick up this one. To my great surprise and delight, on the
other end of the line was the voice of my best friend, Agi.

To give you a little bit of background, Agi and I have
known each other since practically the first day of high
school. We have been in and out of more predicaments
together than most people will see in a lifetime. Although we
were not born of the same blood, we consider each other
sisters, and are even asked by strangers periodically if we
are.

In any event, I don't remember what small talk
transpired between us, but I will never forget the bombshell
news she dropped on me when she told me that the doctors
had discovered she had breast cancer. I must have asked her
if she was sure at least 10 times, along with saying that I
couldn't believe it.

At this point, Agi still didn't know what she was
going to do. This only made it worse for me when we ended
our conversation.

It's a helpless feeling being thousands of miles away
from someone you care so much about, a part of your family,
and not being able to help. I knew she had a wonderful man

in her life, "Bill", and a close knit group of friends to support her, but I could only imagine the worse.

The next phone call I received from Agi was to tell me she was considering choosing the natural route, and was looking into a cleansing program in northern California.

After digesting this information I called Agi back, but all I kept getting was her answering machine. After a week of fruitless calling, I called Debbie, a good friend of ours, to get an update. Debbie told me Agi had gone to California for internal cleansing and education, whereupon we had a lengthy discussion on our grave doubts and concerns over Agi's decision.

I came back to the US in mid-September with great trepidation as to how I was going to find her. She was skinny and I wondered even then if she was doing the right thing. Agi never had a moment of doubt and was filled with so much enthusiasm, so who was I to contribute any doubt.

After a while, **Agi's excitement caught on to all of us.** We looked forward to not only hearing about the kinds of things you don't want to think exists in your body, but also helping Agi with some of the natural treatments involved in her healing.

Looking back, I remember leaving Agi a message trying to convince her to seek conventional medical treatment because I was not about to bury my best friend. Today, over four years after the fact, *I am a true believer in natural healing.*

Linda

I consider Linda to be family. Linda supported me through major transitions in my life.

When my husband and I first met Agi 12 years ago she was like no one we've ever known. She was upbeat, optimistic and totally without inhibition in her enthusiasm for any new undertaking she claimed was hers. Agi was a natural at bringing people together and keeping them in the moment, looking only at what was right, natural and fun.

Then all of a sudden she disappeared... not literally, but to the extent that her contact with friends waned and she withdrew into herself (I realize now it was the time when she went into a deep depression).

To all our great despair she was diagnosed with breast cancer. When a friend gets this kind of news it doesn't just happen to them. It happens to everyone who's close to him or her. How you feel when your friend tells you she was just given the recommendation to have her breast removed...goes beyond thinking.

We cried and Agi prepared for the fate of living without a breast, losing her hair, and all the other horrendous things that they would put her body through. Then all of a sudden, some incredible things started happening to Agi that I couldn't explain. One by one she was put in contact with people who greatly influenced her decision to go with a non-conventional treatment regimen. So in great Agi fashion, she took this decision to heart and trusted God to keep her afloat and jumped in with both feet.

She started juicing, drinking green stuff and went to California to learn about natural healing. When she returned she was full blown into the prospect of healing herself naturally. Again, she was put in touch with people that helped her journey. ***She grew close to God and as she took His hand, she marched on her most important quest thus far.***

And what about the rest of us... her mother, her fiancé, her "best friends?" What were we thinking and how were we reacting? All of the natural healing she was expounding made sense. I am a strong believer in a positive mind and a strong will, but could I give my whole body and soul to the idea? Eating right and healthier, who could oppose that, but what IF it didn't work? The idea of watching her do something that may not produce the results, we all so desperately wanted, was more than I could bear at times.

She started "her program" and was fiercely committed to a lifestyle that was hard and difficult, yet she had a purpose and she was going to succeed.

The cold sheet treatment was quite an experience. I was there with her during the first and second one. I watched and encouraged her to build more and more white blood cells to fight those nasty cancer cells.

It wasn't easy. She sat in a hot bath, drank hot tea, the sweat pouring out of her body, then we wrapped her in an ice soaked sheet and wrapped her in a blanket! Again she drank and drank water while wrapped up. It took a lot out of her. Agi said it was invigorating and she could feel her body was fighting.

Agi continued to do her program. I watched her lose weight and get an incredibly attractive body. I also watched her lose more and more weight until one day I finally said, "Are you sure you're supposed to be this skinny? You look pale and you have dark circles under your eyes. Are you sure you don't want to go for a check up?" She replied, "Before I can completely be healed my body has to be stripped down to bare minimum. I'm loading my body with nutrition and starving this cancer to death."

It's been over four years and *Agi looks great!* She remains convinced she is healed and she certainly appears to be.

What Agi has done for me is show me how strong we humans can be. How it is to dig deep within yourself when faced with your toughest battle. She has surely proven to me, as well as our friends, that allowing God into your heart, having tremendous faith, remaining open and optimistic, eating right and with finding the right natural healing herbs that *miracles do happen!*

Sharon

Sharon is the older sister I never had. She encouraged me through my entire healing journey. Never doubting the positive outcome.

A walking, talking, living miracle of Jesus Christ is what Agi truly is!

I'll never forget the day Agi called and said she had breast cancer. "My God, it's not possible", I cried. I was with her during the biopsy and the radiologist was so positive it was benign.

Almost immediately during the phone call, the Holy Spirit imparted to me that Agi must be saved.

Agi proceeded to tell me, "Here's the deal. The doctors want to cut off my breast, take some lymph nodes and give me chemotherapy." I began sharing information with her about the ancient healing properties of various herbs. I only began reading books on this subject of few weeks prior to her phone call.

I witnessed Agi being led, like a child lost in the forest, by the loving hand of the Lord. She found her way back to the land of the living. It was like her destiny was being unfolded right before my eyes.

God was using me as His vessel to help Agi through her healing journey. First by having me read about natural healing methods two weeks before she told me she had breast cancer and to teach Agi about the Lord through scripture.

I knew it wasn't Agi's time to leave this world. She had a purpose to fulfill. Agi is now a healthy woman with a long life ahead of her. As it says in the Bible: **"All things work together for good for those who love God and are called according to His purpose."**

125

Lidle Café

Cookbook

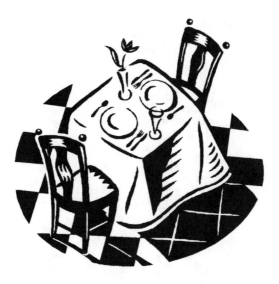

How the Lidle Café came to be...

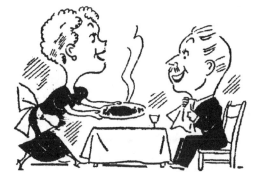

Named after Bill & Agi Lidle
this festive café for two
serves divinely inspired dishes
while enjoying a pines view
our hats off to chef Agi
whose past attempts were "Peeu"
either burnt or too soggy
menu selection was few
her efforts never wavered
as she prayed for the passion to cook
the prayers were soon answered
delicious recipes now appear in this book

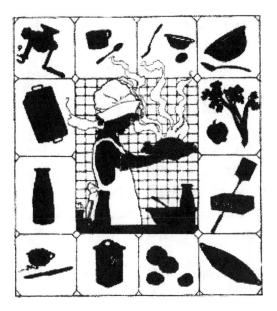

Get your kids involved in helping prepare these recipes. There are products on the market that make interactive cooking with your kids fun. Products like the spiral dicer make zucchini, cucumber, sweet potato and squash look like angel hair pasta. Kids love to play with their food and they'll love angel hair vegetables.

Most of the Lidle Café favorites are festive and colorful...and the flavor...oom good! Who would have thought vegetarian food could taste this good?

When I was first diagnosed with breast cancer my repertoire consisted of a handful of recipes. I just didn't like to cook. My kitchen was bare. Thankfully, friends came to my aid and stocked the kitchen with everything I would need to begin my healing journey.

Two years after the diagnosis, I was well into living a healthy vegetarian lifestyle. By spending so much time preparing fresh juices, I came to appreciate my kitchen. Still I didn't have the passion for learning how to prepare new recipes.

Bill never complained. We ate lots of fresh fruits and vegetables, steamed vegetables and brown rice, potatoes, black beans, salsa, vegetarian chili, garden burgers and lots of Amy's frozen foods.

After a while we got tired of eating the same things and we began to go out to eat. We found a handful of restaurants that we trusted to use fresh ingredients. This too was beginning to get old. More and more often we felt that what we ate at home was better.

Just over a year ago, I did pray for the passion to cook. My prayers were answered almost immediately because I began to try new recipes. Many were good and many were a flop. We always had back up vegetarian chili in the freezer or Amy's frozen pizza.

I picked six recipes as my foundation and built on them. I followed the recipe but added some of my own ingredients and eliminated some. This came to be because every single time I followed a recipe to a tee, it didn't turn out right.

Surprisingly, almost every time I added my own twists the recipe turned out great. So, as the months went on I experimented with many fresh herbs and spices. It was so much fun to see how many different colors the finished piece of artwork would be.

I call my dishes artwork because most of them are so pretty and filled with color. The aroma's that burst forth are indescribable. All of a sudden I was filled with the passion to create new tastes. I even love my pots and pans.

As you try out the recipes in the Lidle Café Cookbook please keep in mind that I'm not the best when it comes to measuring. I gave it my best shot. I trust the recipes as they are written are wonderful.

BE ENCOURAGED to step out of your complacency or comfort zone like I did. Add your own twists to the recipes. Delete or add ingredients. Step out and PLAY......CREATE......BECOME YOUR OWN CHEF...... IT'S FUN!

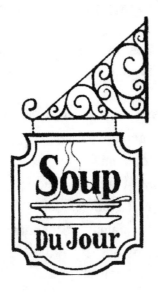

Creamy Corn Chowder

Refreshing Carrot Soup

Potato & Leek Soup

Vegetarian Chili

Five Bean & Barley Soup

Nutritional & Healing Vegetable Broth

Creamy Corn Chowder

When fresh corn is in season, this soup is delicious. Kids will like it because it's sweet.

- ➤ 4 cups fresh corn kernels (about 4 ears of corn)
- ➤ 1 teaspoon ground cumin
- ➤ 2 cups almond milk
- ➤ 2 teaspoons of minced onion
- ➤ Big pinch of Celtic sea salt
- ➤ Big pinch Herbamare Seasoning
- ➤ Few shakes of garlic powder
- ➤ 1 avocado in small chunks

In a blender, combine most of the corn, almond milk, most of the avocado, cumin, and seasonings. Blend well and stir in extra corn. If it's too thick add a little more almond milk. Decorate with a little corn on top with a few avocado chunks.

Lidle Café Twists: Substitute shallots for onions, sprinkle small pieces of red pepper on top with a sprinkle of Hungarian Paprika for garnish. Try it first the way the recipe reads...if it's not to your taste...add your own twists...like jalapeno...sweet basil...even a little curry.

Recipe serves 3-4

Refreshing & Nourishing Carrot Soup

- ➤ 1 cup fresh carrot juice (use a juicer or vita mix)
- ➤ 1/2 -1 avocado
- ➤ 1 teaspoon or more lemon juice
- ➤ 1 clove or more garlic
- ➤ Big pinch Celtic sea salt
- ➤ Big pinch ground cumin
- ➤ Big pinch coriander

In a blender, combine carrot juice and avocado. Add cumin, coriander, lemon juice, salt and garlic. Save a few pieces of avocado to garnish the top of the soup.

Lidle Café Twists: Try adding grated ginger, jalapeno, chopped red and green peppers, thinly sliced celery, sweet basil, corn kernels, bite size chunks of zucchini...even a little curry powder.

I find with carrot soup, most people like a small serving with salad or main course.

Recipe serves 1-2

Potato, Celery & Leek Soup

- 4 or 5 potatoes red or white potatoes, small bite sizes
- 1 sweet potato, small bite sizes (optional)
- 2-4 leeks, sliced thin
- 3 stalks celery sliced thin
- A couple of big pinches of Celtic sea salt
- 2 bay leaves and sweet basil if you have it
- 4-8 cloves garlic minced
- 3 or more tablespoons Herbamare
- 2 or more tablespoon Chik'Nish seasoning

In a medium to large soup pot, add 14 cups of water and bring to almost boil. Turn down to simmer.

In a sauté pan over medium heat, sauté leeks, garlic and celery in a little olive oil about 8 minutes. Add potatoes, salt, leeks, garlic, celery, and sweet potato to simmering water. Bring to a very slow boil for 15 minutes.

After 15 minutes add herbs and spices and cook on simmer to low for another 15-20 mutes. I like the potatoes to be a bit firm.

*Take 1/2 of the soup and place in blender. Blend it up for a minute and put it back with the rest of the soup. This thickens it up. To make creamy soup, pour it all into the blender and blend.

Vegetarian Chili

Everyone loves vegetarian chili. They ask for the recipe all the time, but I've never measured any of the ingredients before, so here it goes. Remember you can always add more or less...to your liking. This chili freezes well. It's always good for a back up.

- ➤ 1 cup pinto beans
- ➤ 1 cup navy beans
- ➤ 1 cup black beans
- ➤ 3 carrots sliced thin
- ➤ 2 white or yellow onions minced
- ➤ 3 green peppers diced
- ➤ 4-5 stalks celery chopped medium
- ➤ 3 zucchini sliced medium
- ➤ 4-6 tablespoons chili powder
- ➤ 3-4 teaspoons Celtic sea salt
- ➤ at least 4 cloves of garlic minced (if you love garlic, leave some extra whole pieces in)
- ➤ 4 or more tablespoons Cumin
- ➤ 4 tablespoons of Turmeric
- ➤ 2 16oz cans of peeled tomatoes
  or 5-7 fresh tomatoes peeled (blanch in boiling water for a minute before peeling)
- ➤ 1 16oz can of tomato puree

Put beans in a bowl and cover with water. Soak overnight. The next day, rinse the beans with water and put them in the big pot you're cooking the chili in. Fill with water (about four inches above beans). Bring to a boil and lower heat to slow cook for one hour (after 30 Minutes, check to see if the water level is ok. If it's cooked down to close to the beans, add a little more.)

When beans are cooked, after one hour there should be 2-3 inches of water over the beans.

While the beans are boiling, skim off the brown residue on top.

A few minutes before the beans have finished cooking cooking, in a sauté pan on medium heat, sauté onions, peppers, celery, zucchini and carrots for 8 minutes. Add these to the beans and water. Add tomatoes and paste at this time too.

Add all of the spices and taste after 30-40 minutes. We like it spicy, so I add extra jalapeno's and chili powder. Simmer another 15-20 minutes. Two hours seems about right for total cooking time.

It seems like during the cooking process the spices are absorbed...that's why I over spice it.

Serves 10-15

Five Bean, Vegetable & Barley Soup

This is one of the Lidle Café favorite soups. I make extra and freeze it. The vegetarian chili and this soup is found in our freezer at all times.

- ➢ 1/2 cup black beans
- ➢ 1/2 cup navy beans
- ➢ 1/2 cup pinto beans
- ➢ 1/2 cup lima beans
- ➢ 1/2 cup lentils
- ➢ 1/2 - 3/4 cup barley
- ➢ 4 stalks celery sliced thin
- ➢ 1 onion minced or 3 shallots
- ➢ 1 green pepper chopped
- ➢ 1 zucchini in bite size pieces
- ➢ 8-10 cloves garlic chopped
- ➢ 2-3 sprigs fresh sweet basil
- ➢ Small handful of parsley (full sprigs)
- ➢ 2 tablespoons garlic powder
- ➢ 2-3 tablespoons Herbamare
- ➢ 2-3 tablespoons cumin
- ➢ 2-3 tablespoons Chik'Nish
- ➢ Celtic sea salt to taste
- ➢ 1 jalapeno chopped (optional) tastes great with!

If you don't have all of the above ingredients it's o.k. It tastes great even without Chik'Nish or Herbamare. You do need cumin. Use your favorite spices.

Pour beans in a large bowl, cover with water and soak overnight. Next day, rinse the beans and put the beans and the barley in the big pot you're using to make the soup. Add water to at least five inches over the top of the beans. They will swell along with the barley.

It shouldn't be too soupy but not too thick either. You can always add more water during the cooking process. It's better to start with too little than too much.

Bring beans and barley to a slow boil for about 50 minutes. While the beans and barley are cooking in a sauté pan on medium heat, sauté the chopped onions, celery, garlic and green peppers.

After 50 minutes add onions, celery, garlic, zucchini, green pepper, sweet basil, parsley and the herbs and spices. Cover and check periodically and taste...you may want to add more seasonings and spices.

Slow cook (not boil) for 1½ hours. The perfect amount of liquid when finished is about 1½ - 2 inches above the ingredients.

Nutritional & Healing Vegetable Broth

- 4 large potato peelings (only peelings)
- 5 stalks of celery cut in a few pieces
- Handful of parsley
- 10-15 cloves garlic whole
- 6 carrot peelings (only peelings)
- Handful of fresh spinach
- Handful of fresh kale and/or chard
- Handful of fresh bok choy, if available
- 4-6 tablespoons Herbamare or your favorite seasoning
- 1 jalapeno chopped
- 1 onion cut in half

In a large soup pot, add all of the above ingredients. Add just enough distilled or purified water to cover the vegetables.

Cover and cook on very low for 1 1/2 hours. Don't bring it to a boil, not even a slow boil.

Strain and drink warm or cold. Nutritional broth will keep in the refrigerator, for three to four days. It also freezes well.

Nutritional broth is cleansing and has an alkalizing effect on the body and is rich with minerals. It's very healing to drink during the flu season.

144

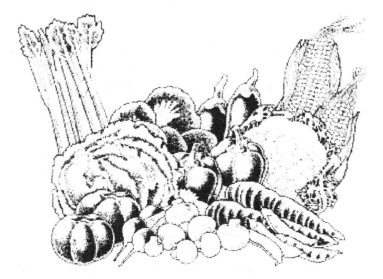

Lidle Café Vegetable Specialties

Potato Casserole Surprise

Creamy Vegetables & Rice

Agi's Signature Vegetable Paté

Seared Tomato & Cauliflower

Beets, Raisins & Carrots

Spicy Green Beans & Garlic Mashed Potatoes

Potato Casserole Surprise

I created this dish about a year and a half ago, just before I prayed for the passion to cook. It was among the few things, to my SURPRISE that turned out. Men really like this recipe.

- ➤ 5 potatoes peeled and cubed in bite size pieces
- ➤ 2 stalks of celery cut thin
- ➤ 1 zucchini cut thin
- ➤ Handful of cauliflower cut in bite sizes
- ➤ 1/2 red pepper chopped
- ➤ 1/2- 1 onion chopped
- ➤ 4 or more cloves of garlic chopped
- ➤ 2 or more tablespoons of Herbamare
- ➤ Big pinch of Paprika (optional)
- ➤ 2-4 tablespoons of olive oil (more makes a little sauce, less is probably better for your health)
- ➤ Big pinch of sweet basil or little bit of rosemary
- ➤ Jalapeno chopped (optional)

In a mixing bowl, add all of the above ingredients except olive oil. Add olive oil and mix. Pour into a baking dish and bake at 375° for one hour. After about 30 minutes I stir it up a bit. Hint: The more fresh herbs and spice the better. If you think you've over done the spices it's the perfect amount.

Serves 2-3

Creamy Vegetables and Brown Rice

This is another dish I created on a whim. I had left over Creamy Dill & Sweet Basil Dressing, so I decided to sauté up some vegetables and left over brown rice. Just before it was done, I added the dressing.

- ➢ 1 medium zucchini cut into very small pieces
- ➢ 2 shallots or 1/2 red onion minced
- ➢ 2 cloves of garlic minced
- ➢ A few shakes of Herbamare or sea salt
- ➢ A few shakes of Italian seasoning
- ➢ 2 tablespoons of fresh chopped basil (optional)
- ➢ 1 1/2 cups cooked brown rice

In a sauté pan over medium heat, sauté onions, garlic and 1 1/2 cups of cooked brown rice (already prepared or leftover from the night before). Let it get almost burnt at the bottom...but don't burn it.

Stir in the rest of the ingredients and cook for a few more minutes. About a minute before it's done pour about 1/2 to 1 cup of the Creamy Dill & Sweet Basil Dressing over the top. Stir and let simmer for a minute or two.

Serve with a salad made of sliced cucumbers, onions, and red peppers mixed with the Creamy Dill & Sweet Basil Dressing. Serves 2-3

Agi's Signature Vegetable Paté

This paté is a winner. For this recipe a Champion Juicer is best. It will work in a Cuisinart, but the texture will be different.

> - 1 cup raw almonds, soaked in water overnight
> - 1/4 cup ground flax seeds (optional)
> - 1/2 each, red and green or yellow bell pepper
> - 1-2 cloves garlic
> - 1/2 of a sweet potato
> - 1-2 carrots
> - 1 shallot or 1/4 - 1/2 of an onion
> - 2-3 tablespoons of Herbamare
> - 2 tablespoons of Chik'Nish
> - 1 teaspoon coriander

Run all of the ingredients except the flax seeds through the juicer with the BLANK SCREEN on. Put a small amount of nuts in first and push through, then follow it with a piece of carrot or another vegetable. If you put too many nuts in at a time, it will clog up the juicer and cause it to overheat.

Paté is wonderful on crackers or as a sandwich spread. Refrigerate, keeps fresh for 4 days.

Hint: Chop up fresh sweet basil about 2 tablespoons and mix it in at the end. Serves 7-10

Pan Seared Tomato and Cauliflower

This festive vegetable side dish is terrific over a bit of soy or rice pasta...or brown rice.

Chef William, in Phoenix, has been a great inspiration for me to dive in and create sautéed vegetable side dishes. This is one of Chef Williams creations with the Lidle Café Twist.

- ➤ Handful of cauliflower cut into bite sized pieces
- ➤ 2 tomatoes cored, remove the center and cut into 6 wedges
- ➤ 3 tablespoons shallots minced
- ➤ 1-2 cloves of garlic minced
- ➤ 2 teaspoons olive oil
- ➤ 2 tablespoon fresh chopped basil or oregano
- ➤ 4-6 Shakes of Chefs All Purpose Blend
- ➤ 1 teaspoon coriander

First, steam the cauliflower for a few minutes. If you don't have time, just cut them up into really small thin pieces so they cook faster. In a sauté pan over medium to high heat, cook tomatoes without olive oil for 2-3 minutes. Cooking tomatoes without oil caramelizes them and turns them alkaline.

Add olive oil, cauliflower, herbs and spices and cook over medium heat for 5-8 minutes. Just a minute before it's ready, add a splash of red wine. Serves 2

Beets, Raisins & Carrots

This is another of Chef Williams inspired recipes. The raisins give it an unusually good taste.

- ➤ 1-2 grated beets
- ➤ 1 grated carrot
- ➤ Chop some of the beet greens, stems and leaves
- ➤ 1/4 cup raisins
- ➤ 2 teaspoons shallots or red onions chopped
- ➤ 1 clove garlic minced
- ➤ 2 tablespoons of olive oil (not extra virgin)
- ➤ 2 teaspoons balsamic vinegar
- ➤ A splash of red wine (optional)

In a sauté pan over medium heat, sauté the beet stems, garlic, shallots and oil for one minute or two.

Add beets, carrots and raisins and sauté for a few minutes longer. Add beet leaves and toss lightly.

Add vinegar and a splash of wine and sauté for another minute.

Serves 2

Spicy Green Beans & Garlic Mashed Potatoes

Not long ago, Bill asked me to make him a Turkey Breast. I did, and decided to make it a Thanksgiving meal. This was just one week after the bombing of the World Trade Center Towers and the Pentagon.

We felt led to give thanks to God and all people who united to help each other. Bill and I were grateful for what we had.

As I flipped through the channels that morning, to watch the different perspectives of the tragedy...I landed on the cooking channel. There was Martha Stewart, preparing these wonderful beans. I followed her recipe with a few twists of my own. They turned out great!

➤ A couple of handfuls of fresh long green beans cut in half with the ends cut off
➤ 1/2 red pepper chopped, small pieces
➤ 1/2 zucchini julienne strips
➤ 2 cloves garlic minced
➤ 1 onion chopped
➤ A pinch of crushed red pepper
➤ A handful of sweet basil sprigs (stems & leaves)
➤ 3-4 shakes of Herbamare
➤ 2-3 tablespoons olive oil

In a large sauté pan over medium heat, sauté onions and garlic in olive oil for one minute. Add green beans, stir and cook on low heat for 15 minutes.

Add the zucchini, red peppers, crushed red peppers sweet basil and spices. Mix together, cover and cook over low heat for 15 more minutes.

Cover let stand for a few minutes. To cook green beans faster, steam them for 10 minutes or cook them in a little water for 10 minutes.   Serves 2-3

Garlic Mashed Potatoes

Peel 3 potatoes and cut into chunks. Place in water and bring to boil. Add a little sea salt to the water. Boil for 20 minutes. While the potatoes are boiling, peel and mince 4-6 cloves of garlic and brown in a little olive oil until roasted.

After 20 minutes, drain the water off the potatoes leaving just a little. Add about 2 tablespoons of almond or rice milk. Add a little Herbamare or sea salt (a small piece of organic butter is good) and the roasted garlic and mash.

Serve the Spicy Green Beans on top of the garlic mashed potatoes...yum! A meat eater may not even notice there's no meat.

SANDWICHES

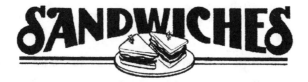

and Wraps

Lidle Café Veggie Sandwich

Roasted Eggplant, Corn and Zucchini Wrap

Garden Salad Wrap

Breakfast Wrap

Mexican Rancheros Wrap

Creamy Dill & Sweet-Basil Wrap Dressing

Hot Pepper Cashew Cheese Spread

"Almonnaise" -Mayonnaise Substitute

Mustard Sauce

Lidle Café Veggie Sandwich

Veggie sandwiches are easy to make and great to take to work. They give you energy instead of taking it. If more people ate veggie sandwiches at lunch, they wouldn't need the extra café mocha to stay awake in the afternoon.

Hummus & Avocado Veggie Sandwich

- A few thin slices of tomato
- 1/4 avocado mashed with a fork
- 4 thin slices of cucumber
- A thin slice of onion (optional)
- A few sprouts
- Hummus to spread on the bread
- A dab of mustard sauce
- A few sprinkles of sunflower seeds
- Ezekiel bread or Whole wheat pita

Vegetable Paté Sandwich

- Vegetable Paté spread on bread
- A few thin slices of red or yellow pepper
- 4 thin slices of cucumber
- 1/4 avocado mashed with fork
- Mustard Sauce
- Leaf of Romaine lettuce
- On Ezekiel bread, cabbage or lettuce leaves

Roasted Eggplant, Corn & Zucchini Wrap

- ➤ A handful of eggplant cubed, small bite sizes
- ➤ 1 corn on the cob (cut kernels off the cob)
- ➤ 1/2 zucchini julienned
- ➤ 1 tomato cored and cut into chunks
- ➤ 1/2 onion thin long slices
- ➤ 1 clove garlic minced
- ➤ 4 lettuce leaves torn in small pieces
- ➤ Add Herbamare or your favorite seasoning
- ➤ Jalapeno chopped (optional)
- ➤ Large whole wheat or spinach tortilla

In a sauté pan in-between medium to high heat, roast the corn kernels until they have some brown spots on corn or the bottom of the pan turns brown from the milk escaping the corn.

Add tomato and cook for another minute or two. Add the rest of the ingredients with a small bit of olive oil. Sauté for a few more minutes. In a bowl, mix the vegetables with the lettuce. For a twist: Add salad dressing to the filling before wrapping it up.   Serves 2

How to wrap your filling: Heat the tortilla for a minute in a pan or over the burner. Lay it flat and add filling to the 1/3 side of the tortilla closest to you. Begin to wrap. As you make one complete turn, tuck in the ends and continue to roll it up.

Garden Salad Wrap

This is a wonderful way to eat your salad. Your kids may even eat salad this way, because it's covered up by the wrap.

*If you prefer to eat a completely uncooked wrap, substitute cabbage leaves and lettuce leaves in the place of the tortilla.

> ➢ 1 tomato chopped into small pieces
> ➢ 1/2 cucumber diced
> ➢ 1 avocado diced
> ➢ A little chopped onion (optional)
> ➢ 1/2 yellow or green bell pepper diced
> ➢ 5-8 lettuce leaves torn into small pieces
> ➢ A pinch of fresh basil
> ➢ Sprouts
> ➢ Hummus to spread on tortilla
> ➢ Large whole wheat or spinach tortilla

In a bowl, mix the above ingredients and spoon into a tortilla with hummus spread on it...and wrap it up.

Lidle Café Twist: Pour Creamy Dill & Sweet Basil Dressing...or Dip your wrap into the Hot Pepper Cheese Spread...or spread the Cheese Spread on the tortilla before filling it...CedarBrook avocado dressing...or your favorite Italian dressing. Serves 1

Breakfast Wrap

Wraps are the easiest and fasted foods to prepare for even the pickiest of eaters.

- ➢ 1 package firm organic tofu
- ➢ 1/2 - 1 onion chopped
- ➢ 1/2 of a small zucchini julienned
- ➢ 1 corn on the cob (cut kernels off)
- ➢ 1/3 of a red, green or yellow bell pepper (chopped) Mix all three for more color
- ➢ A teaspoon of Turmeric and a few shakes of Herbamare
- ➢ 1 clove of garlic or a few shakes of garlic powder
- ➢ A little olive oil
- ➢ Large whole wheat or spinach tortilla

Cut the kernels off the fresh corn. Don't cut to close to the core. In a medium sauté pan over medium heat with no oil, cook the corn about 3 minutes. Add onions and garlic and continue cooking for 2 minutes.

Add tofu and turmeric, mix together for 3 more minutes (mash tofu with a fork and it will look like scrambled eggs). Add the rest of the ingredients including spices for 3-4 more minutes. If you prefer vegetables more cooked add an additional 4 minutes.

Spoon into the tortilla, wrap it up and enjoy. Serves 2

Mexican Rancheros Wrap

- 3-4 organic eggs scrambled
- 1/2 onion chopped
- 1/2 small zucchini diced bite sizes
- 2 cloves garlic minced
- 1/2 green pepper chopped
- 1/2 jalapeno minced
- 3 or more tablespoons of salsa
- A few pinches of cilantro
- Large whole wheat or spinach tortilla

In a sauté pan over medium heat, sauté onions and garlic for 5 minutes. Add peppers, zucchini, and jalapeno. Cook 2 minutes. Stir often. Fold in the eggs and add salsa, spices and cilantro. Cook until eggs are done to your liking.

Wrap up the filling in a warmed sprouted or whole wheat, or spinach tortilla.

Rancheros wrap is delicious accompanied by a side of refried beans.

Serves 2

Creamy Dill & Sweet Basil Wrap Dressing

This is a wonderful dressing. We use at the Lidle Café in the creamy vegetables and brown rice recipe. Try it in any of the wraps. It's especially good used as a dipping sauce for wraps without dressing inside.

- ➤ 1 box silken tofu
- ➤ 1/2 cup almond milk
- ➤ 1/4 cup water
- ➤ 3 tablespoons fresh squeezed lemon
- ➤ 1 green bell pepper cut in four
- ➤ 1 clove fresh garlic or 1 teaspoon garlic powder
- ➤ 1 teaspoon onion powder
- ➤ 2-3 teaspoons dill
- ➤ 2 big pinches of fresh sweet basil
- ➤ 2 tablespoon Italian seasoning or oregano
- ➤ 1 tablespoon Herbamare

Put the tofu, water and one half of the almond milk in the blender or vita mix and blend for two minutes. Add the rest of the ingredients and the remaining almond milk and blend until creamy and smooth.

If it's too thick for your taste add a little more almond milk.

Hot Pepper Cashew Cheese
Spread or Dip

- ➤ 1 cup water
- ➤ 1 cup raw cashews
- ➤ 3 tablespoons brewer's yeast
- ➤ 1 teaspoon onion powder
- ➤ Juice of 1/2 lemon
- ➤ 3-4 tablespoons fresh green chilies or 1 small jar of green chilies
- ➤ 1/4 teaspoon sea salt
- ➤ 1/4 fresh red pepper or green pepper
- ➤ 1 jalapeno
- ➤ 1 teaspoon garlic powder or 1 clove garlic

Blend all ingredients in blender until smooth and place in refrigerator for 15 minutes. Hot Pepper Cheese Spread is really good on sandwiches, toast, baked potato and cut up carrot and celery sticks. Will keep in refrigerator for 3 to 4 days.

Lidle Twist: Try adding fajita or taco seasoning in place of the jalapeno.

Almonnaise
Mayonnaise Substitute

I made this for the first time, just a few months ago, and it almost tastes like mayonnaise.

- ➢ 1/2 cup blanched almonds
- ➢ 1/2 cup water or almond milk
- ➢ 1 clove garlic
- ➢ 1/2 teaspoon Herbamare or herb seasoning
- ➢ 1/2 teaspoon sea salt
- ➢ 3 tablespoons fresh lemon juice
- ➢ 1 cup olive oil (I don't use extra virgin in this recipe)

To blanch almonds, place almonds in boiling water for 1 minute. Strain off water and hold almonds between your fingers and squeeze. The skin just pops off. Kids love to pop the skins off.

Place almonds in the blender with water and blend for a few minutes. Add the rest of the ingredients using only one half of the oil at first. Blend for a few minutes and slowly add the remaining oil. If it's still too thick add a little more almond milk.

Lidle Café Twist: Add jalapeno, cayenne pepper, fajita seasoning, and chives, even dill. Stays fresh in refrigerator for 4 days.

MUSTARD SAUCE

- ➢ 1/2 cup mustard seed powder
- ➢ 2oz raw apple cider vinegar
- ➢ 1oz water

Mix the vinegar and water together and slowly add to the mustard seed powder. To make Honey Mustard add a little bit of honey. Add cayenne or jalapeno to make it hot mustard sauce.

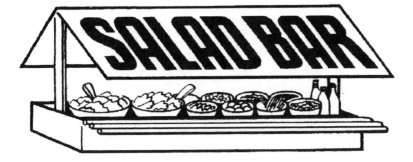

Lidle Café Festive Garden Salad with
Olive Oil & Vinegar Dressing

Medley Crunch Vinegar-Free Salad

Ginger, Beet and Carrot Vinaigrette

CedarBrook Avocado Dressing

Green Olive Dressing

Lidle Café Festive Garden Salad

I discovered the secret to a good salad, using oil & vinegar or oil & lemon is to LET THE CUT VEGGIES MARINATE IN THE DRESSING FOR AT LEAST 10-15 MINUTES.

In a salad bowl add:

- 1-3 cloves garlic chopped or pressed
- 1 leek, 1 shallot or red onion sliced thin
- About 6 or more tablespoons olive oil
- 2 tablespoons raw apple cider vinegar or the juice of 1 lemon
- 1 tablespoon balsamic Vinegar, optional
- Herbamare a few shakes
- Pinch of sea salt
- 1 cucumber sliced very thin
- 1/2 green pepper chopped
- 1/2 yellow pepper chopped
- 1 tomato bite size pieces
- 1 small handful cauliflower tops, almost shaved, it's like feta cheese
- Romaine lettuce

Now, let it stand and marinate (stir it around a few times) for at least 10 minutes. Wash and tear apart the lettuce. I find more people like lettuce torn up into little pieces better than big awkward pieces. Mix together and sprinkle raw sunflower seeds on top.

Medley Crunch Vinegar-Free Salad

The colors in this salad make it a piece of artwork. Before eating this salad, take a minute to appreciate the colors. This is a unique salad because there is no lettuce in it.

My passion for creative cooking continues, because of the beautiful colors...that result in combining different vegetables. It also brings out the kid in me. I'm free and uninhibited when I cook!

- ➢ 1 cucumber sliced thin
- ➢ 1/2 orange bell pepper chopped
- ➢ 1/2 yellow bell pepper chopped
- ➢ 1/2 red onion sliced in long thin strips
- ➢ 1 clove garlic chopped or pressed
- ➢ A small handful of fresh sweet basil chopped
- ➢ A few shakes of Herbamare
- ➢ A few big pinches of fresh or dried oregano
- ➢ Olive oil
- ➢ Juice of 1 lemon

Put all the above ingredients into a large salad bowl. Add enough Olive Oil to vegetables to coat them well, with a little left on the bottom. Mix well and let stand for at least 10-15 minutes before serving. This salad is the perfect compliment to Pistachio Pesto Pasta.

Ginger, Beet & Carrot Vinaigrette

This is a Chef William creation, and it's wonderful. Many of us want to eat more beets, we just don't know how to fix them. Here's a fast and easy way.

- ➢ 6 ounces beets grated
- ➢ 2 ounces beet greens, stem diced, leaves julienned
- ➢ 1 carrot grated
- ➢ 3-4 radish grated
- ➢ 1 tablespoon ginger root peeled & grated
- ➢ 3 teaspoons shallots chopped
- ➢ 2 tablespoons olive oil

In medium sauté pan over medium heat, pour the olive oil in one side of the pan forming a puddle. Place the ginger in the oil for thirty seconds or until slightly brown.

Add the beet stems and leaves with the garlic and shallots. Add carrot, radish and beets and sauté for two and a half minutes.

Pour dressing on top of baby lettuce, warm napa cabbage and bok choy. Mix together and enjoy!

Optional Twist: At the last minute splash a small bit of white wine or apple cider vinegar.   Serves 2

CedarBrook Avocado Dressing

Put 1 cup of water in blender and add:
- ➢ 3/4 cups raw cashews

Add 1 more cup of water and add:
- ➢ 1/4 cup raw sesame seeds
- ➢ 1/2 avocado
- ➢ 1-2 cloves garlic
- ➢ Pinch of cayenne
- ➢ 1 teaspoon sea salt
- ➢ 1 teaspoon onion powder
- ➢ Juice of one lemon

Blend all ingredients 1-2 minutes, until smooth.

The Lidle Café Twist: Add 1/2 cucumber and sweet basil or add green pepper and jalapeno. If you don't have sesame seeds or cashews, raw almonds work really well. Try doing the recipe with almond milk. Add dill or any other of your favorite herbs. If limes are juicy, squeeze some juice into the mixture.

*Make the dressing a little thicker by adding more avocado or nuts and the result is a fabulous dip for vegetables.

Green Olive Dressing

For olive lovers, this one's a winner! I first tasted this dressing at CedarBrook. Personally, I don't like olives but everyone who did loved it. So, if you or someone you know loves olives, this dressing is super simple to make.

- ➢ 1 can green pitted olives including juice
- ➢ Juice of one lemon
- ➢ 1 small clove garlic
- ➢ 1/2 avocado optional

Put all ingredients in the blender. Blend until Smooth. You may want to add some of your favorite spices... possibly Italian.

CedarBrook Potato Salad

This potato salad is better than potato salad made with mayonnaise. It's simply delicious.

- ➢ 1 full recipe of Almonnaise
- ➢ 10 medium, diced cooked potatoes (boil 20 min.)
- ➢ 1/4 cup celery chopped
- ➢ 1/4 cup drained olives chopped
- ➢ 1/2 red onion chopped
- ➢ 1 tablespoon Celtic sea salt
- ➢ 2 cloves garlic pressed
- ➢ 1 teaspoon dill
- ➢ 1/3 cup green pepper chopped
- ➢ 1 teaspoon Herbamare with a pinch of cayenne pepper
- ➢ 3-5 radishes thinly sliced
- ➢ Add turmeric 1/4 teaspoon at a time to get desired color

For a zesty flavor add a little mustard sauce. For a sweeter flavor add a little Honey.

Put all ingredients in a bowl and mix well. If it looks too dry add more Almonnaise.

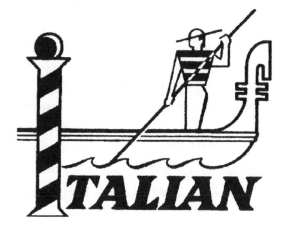

ITALIAN

Sweet Basil & Kalamata Olive Marinara Sauce
Cooked & Uncooked Versions

Pistachio Pesto Pasta

Sweet Basil & Kalamata Olive Marinara

Simple, Simple, Simple....to prepare. This Marinara can be eaten uncooked and cooked. The recipe below is for both versions. For the cooked version, simply heat the marinara for a few minutes.

This recipe is PERFECT for the person who enjoys eating more uncooked foods, while at the same time serving it cooked to other members of the family who prefer it cooked.

- ➢ 3 ounces of sun-dried Tomatoes
- ➢ 4 fresh tomatoes
- ➢ 1/4 cup onion chopped
- ➢ 2-3 cloves of Garlic chopped
- ➢ 1/4 cup Kalamata olives pitted
- ➢ 1/2 cup or more fresh sweet basil chopped or 2 tablespoons dried basil
- ➢ 1/4 cup fresh oregano chopped or 2 tablespoons dried oregano

Pre-soak sun-dried tomatoes in water for a few hour before preparing recipe. Drain the tomatoes and put in food processor with all the above ingredients. Blend in until desired consistency. Marina is perfect over uncooked angel hair - zucchini, sweet potato, squash and cucumber. Kids love it. Or try the marinara over brown rice spaghetti or organic soy pasta.

172

Pistachio Pesto Pasta

"This is one of the best meals we had in a long time", Bill said after he finished his third serving. "What do you mean a long time", I answered. I thought my creative cooking has improved greatly. He explained his compliment by telling me it tasted like a gourmet dinner.

It took me about six attempts making Pistachio Pesto Pasta, until I finally figured out what it was missing – Fresh Basil and Oregano. Don't get discouraged if it doesn't turn out perfect the first time. Keep trying because it's worth it.

* Pistachio Pesto Pasta is perfectly matched with the "Medley Crunch Vinegar Free Salad." Serve together on the same plate. Let the flavors mingle.

- ➤ 3/4 cup raw pistachios
- ➤ 1 or more cloves of garlic (start with one)
- ➤ Small handful of fresh basil
- ➤ A few big pinches of fresh oregano or a big pinch of dried oregano
- ➤ A big pinch of fresh parsley
- ➤ Olive oil (I don't use Extra Virgin Olive oil in this recipe because the taste is too strong, it may be fine for you)

- ➤ 1 tablespoons of dried Italian seasoning if you don't have any fresh herbs
- ➤ 2 tablespoons of dried pesto seasoning if you don't have any fresh herbs
- ➤ 16 oz of corn quinoa elbow pasta or soy pasta

Grind the pistachios in a food processor until the mix is coarse but fine (not powder). Empty into the bowl you're going to use to serve the pasta in. Place the fresh herbs and garlic into the processor and chop. Add to the pistachios.

Add the rest of the herbs and mix. Pour enough olive oil to this mixture so it's kind of creamy, with a little olive oil showing in the pesto. If it clumps together it's too dry. You're going to mix it in the pasta, so it has to be a little oily. Start with about 5 tablespoons of olive oil. Add more if it's too dry.

We use corn quinoa elbow pasta. Don't over cook the pasta, it should be a little firm when finished. Angel hair pasta doesn't work well. Soy pasta would be good too. Shorter pastas work best (penne).

16oz of corn quinoa pasta works best. Serve as soon as you mix the pasta into the pesto, because it gets cold quickly. About the only time we eat cheese is with Pesto Pasta. Shave a little Parmesan and sprinkle on top. Serves 2-3

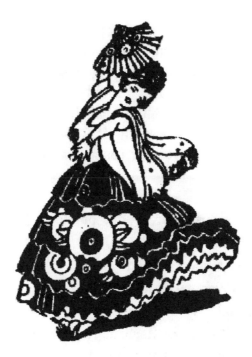

Lidle Café
Specialty of the House

Tortilla Española

Tortilla Española

Just before visiting Spain this past summer, I happened to turn on the Food Network. To my benefit, there was a beautiful young Spanish woman touring Spain and showing off the fabulous foods of the different regions. Tortilla Española was one of them. This is a staple breakfast for many of the local residents. They serve it at room temperature (I prefer it hot).

- ➢ 2 large russet or 3 white potatoes
- ➢ 5 organic eggs
- ➢ 1/2 -1 onion chopped
- ➢ 1-3 cloves garlic minced
- ➢ Olive oil
- ➢ 1-2 tablespoons Herbamare or your favorite seasoning or some sea salt

Peel and cut the potatoes into small pieces. Boil in water for 20 minutes and drain. In a large sauté pan on medium heat, sauté onions and garlic for 8 minutes. While garlic and onions are cooking, scramble the eggs and add the spices.

Crush up the potatoes a bit with a fork so there's still some small pieces, but most of it is kind of mashed up. Add potatoes to the onions and garlic and mix...then add the eggs.

Let it cook for a few minutes...after about 2 minutes use a spatula to separate some of the inside so the uncooked egg can get closer to the bottom of the pan and cook a little. After about 3-4 minutes use the spatula to loosen up the bottom of the mixture. At this point it should look 75% done and somewhat formed.

Remove the pan from the stove and place a plate over the top of the pan...FLIP it upside down holding the plate firmly in place under the pan...shake the pan a bit to loosen the Tortilla Española.

Once it's come out onto the plate, slide it back into the pan and continue to cook for 3-5 more minutes.

It may turn out a little dry your first time or it may turn out perfect. If it falls apart a bit, just reform it in the pan...it will remold itself instantly.

If, when you flip it onto the plate and the pan looks too dry, just add a bit of olive oil to the pan and let it heat up before returning the Tortilla Española back in.

When it's finished it will look like a round cake mold. Slide it onto a plate and let it stand a minute to firm up. Cut into wedges and serve warm or hot. At the Lidle Café, we serve it with Ezekiel Toast and Fresh Fruit.

Lidle Café Twist: To spice it up add: chopped green chili's, jalapeno, fajita or taco spice. Serves 3-4

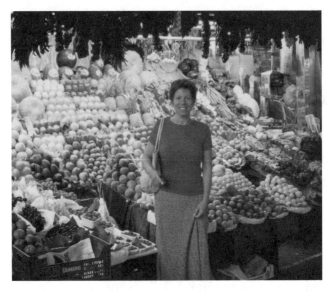

Augis new.tif

The "Mercat de Sant Josep" market in Barcelona, Spain is like no other I've ever visited. It was huge! The local people come to this market each morning to buy fresh produce, fresh herbs, nuts and seeds, fish, poultry, meat, eggs and candy. Bill and I spent three days in Barcelona this summer and had breakfast at this market each morning. Tortilla Española was the first dish I sampled. Accompanying the Tortilla Española was a delicious cup of café con leche. I savored both tastes as long as I could. After breakfast, the indescribably fantastic smells of fresh baked breads and pastries lured us to buy a loaf of bread, almond croissant, and a Spanish donut. Exploring Barcelona while nibbling on these taste treats is a memory I'll never forget. In Europe, Bill and I sample just about everything, except for beef.

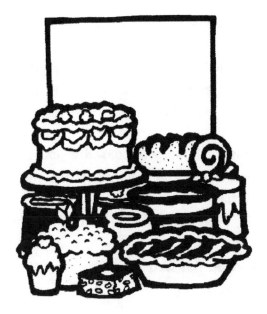

Guilt-Free Desserts

Zesty Lemon Pudding

No-Bake Apple Pie

Orange-Date Dessert Bars

Fruit Fondue

Energy Candy

Zesty Lemon Pudding

Zesty Lemon Pudding

Once you've past the few contemplative bites you'll agree this pudding is good...really good. The texture is hearty, yet creamy.

- ➤ 1 cup raw cashews pre-soaked 8 hours
- ➤ 6 dates pre-soaked 8 hours, pitted and cut into small pieces
- ➤ 1 lemon, peeled, seeded and cut into chunks
- ➤ Juice of 1 lemon
- ➤ 1 tablespoon flaxseed oil
- ➤ Maple syrup
- ➤ Almond milk

In a blender, combine cashews and lemon juice. Blend until smooth. Add lemon pieces, dates and flaxseed oil. Blend until smooth. Taste and if it's too tart for your taste, add a little maple syrup. If it's not tart enough add more pieces of lemon and lemon juice. If it's too thick, add a little almond milk.

Lidle Café Twist: Melt a handful of carob chips and swirl on top of pudding and/or fresh raspberries.

Eat within 4 hours. Serves 3-5

No-Bake Apple Pie

This recipe is an inspiration from Tanya Ferguson who is a 100 percent raw foodist. When she made apple pie for me the first time, I couldn't believe it was so good.

The recipe originally called for dates in the crust, but I don't care for dates, so I put in soaked dried apricots instead. I also love coriander, so I put it in for an extra zing.

CRUST

- 1/2 cup dried un-sulfured apricots, pre-soak in water at least 4 hours
- 2 cups raw almonds
- 3 tablespoons ground flaxseed (optional, highly recommended
- 1/4 cup of raisins, pre-soaked in water, 2 hours
- A few big pinches of unsweetened coconut (optional)
- A big pinch of grated lemon peel

Blend in food processor, work into dough and press into pie plate or two.

FILLING

- 8-10 apples (Granny Smith are good)
- 3/4 cup raisins, pre-soak in water 4 hours
- 1/4 - 1/2 cup fresh apricots or dried apricots, pre-soaked for 4 hours
- 2-4 teaspoons cinnamon
- 1/2 - 1 teaspoon allspice
- A few shakes of coriander
- A few pinches of grated lemon peel

Core and chop apples into bite size pieces. You can peel the apples or leave the peel on.

Take half the apples and the rest of the ingredients and spices, including a few teaspoons of water from the raisins, and mix in food processor. Applesauce consistency or a little chunkier is good.

Set aside and mix the rest of the apples in food processor leaving some chunks for texture. Mix together with the first batch and pour into pie shells.

Lidle Café Twist: Substitute raw pistachios for the almonds. You can use more or less apples...eliminate the apricots if you choose...try fresh peaches and apples. Create your own signature apple pie.

Orange-Date Dessert Bars

Another easy dessert to prepare. These bars are great to take to work, and give your kids for lunch, or breakfast or after dinner.

This is one of my favorite recipes from The Raw Gourmet. It's a great foundation to add your own twists.

CRUST

- 2 cups raw almonds, pecans or walnuts (or try a mixture of all three and a little pistachio)
- 1 cup oat flour
- A pinch of coriander
- 4 tablespoons maple syrup

FILLING

- 2 cups pitted dates, pre-soak 30-60 minutes
- 3 tablespoons water
- Juice and zest (grated rind) of a large orange

Juice the orange and soak the dates in the juice and water.

For crust: Place nuts in food processor and mix until coarsely ground. Add oat flour and pulse to mix. Add coriander and syrup, one tablespoon at a time until mixture holds together.

Press 1/2 of the crust into a lightly oiled pan.

For the filling: In the food processor, combine the dates, the water they soaked in, and orange zest. Puree until smooth.

Spread the date mixture over the crust. Crumble the remaining crust over the top. Press the top crumble lightly into the filling and smooth out the best you can.

*To make oat flour, place whole, raw oat berries or oat grouts in an electric seed grinder. Grind to make flour, and sift any hard bits.

Lidle Café Twist: Fold in fresh raspberries or strawberries into the filling. Add pre-soaked dried apricots, cranberries, blueberries to the filling. Add carob chips to the crust and a little coconut.

Be creative...play...have fun and create your own version.

Serves 6-10

Fruit Fondue

Fruit Fondue is a fast, easy and fun treat. Kids will love it. It may be a way to get them to eat more fruit. If your kids say "Yuk" at carob chips, tell them they're chocolate chips. Or better yet, don't even tell them until they're sold on it.

- ➢ 1 banana sliced in 1/4 inch pieces
- ➢ 10 strawberries left whole
- ➢ 1 apple cut into wedges
- ➢ 1 orange separate slices
- ➢ 1 or more cups melted carob chips

Melt the carob chips in a fondue pot or on top of the stove on low heat. Pour the sauce into a fun dipping bowl and watch excitement begin.

Put some un-sweetened shredded coconut in a little bowl and dip the fruit into the carob sauce and then into the coconut.

Energy Candy

Another recipe your kids will like. Energy candy is great to take to work. Take some on your next trip.

Energy Candy can be made with or without nuts.

- ➢ 1/3 cup dates
- ➢ 1/3 cup raisins
- ➢ 1/4 cup raw sunflower seeds
- ➢ 1/4 cup raw pumpkin seeds
- ➢ 1/4 cup raw almonds
- ➢ 1/4 cup raw cashews
- ➢ 1/4 cup un-sulfured dried apricots
- ➢ 3-4 prunes
- ➢ 3 tablespoons ground flaxseed
- ➢ 1/2 cup unsweetened coconut
- ➢ 1/4 cup raw carob chips or 3 tablespoons carob powder

Put all the ingredients, except carob chips, in food processor and mix until you can form a ball. Fold in carob chips. Form into balls the size of a walnut.

Roll the balls in shredded coconut. You can use as many or as few of the ingredients as you like. It's a shame Girl Scouts didn't sell these candies instead of the cookies many of us overindulge in.

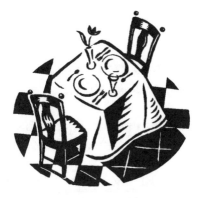

Thank you for giving our Lidle Café favorites a try. I hope they turned out great! If not, I encourage you to keep trying. Remember, Agi wasn't always the chef she is today. If she can do it, so can you.

Agi's husband, Bill

We knew Agi when all she knew how to make were peppered pork chops. We could hardly eat them, but we did to make her feel good.

Our good friends, Bill & Linda

I never imagined Agi would be a cook! She was so awkward in the kitchen. I'm so proud of her.

Agi's mother, Klara

Bibliography and Suggested Reading

Paavo Airola, ND, Ph.D., **How to Get Well** (Health Plus Publishers, Phoenix, Arizona, 1975).

Dr. Richard Schulze, **Patient Handbook** (Dr. Schulze's School of Natural Healing, Santa Monica, California, 1995).

John R. Christopher, ND, M.H., **Dr. Christopher's Three-Day Cleansing Program, Mucusless Diet and Herbal Combinations** (Christopher Publications, Springville, Utah, 1996).

Dr. N.W. Walker, D.Sc., **Become Younger** Norwalk Press, 1995.

Lindsey Duncan, C.N., **Internal Detoxification**, as quoted in the Healthy & Natural Journal, October 1994.

Jethro Kloss, **Back to Eden,** (Back to Eden Books Publishing Company, Loma Linda, California, 1997).

Tonita d'Raye, **FOOD ENZYMES For Vibrant Health and Increased Longevity** (Awieca Inc., 1998).

About the Author

Agi Lidle is a certified herbalist and a graduate of the School of Natural Healing, founded by the esteemed John R. Christopher. She has previously authored the book, "What Will You Do?" and publishes a quarterly newsletter entitled, "The Healing VOICE."

She developed the "Fresh Start Program" and teaches classes designed to guide her students into living a healthier lifestyle. Agi elaborates on the natural health principles described in the book, "Triumph Over Cancer", while demonstrating easy to prepare healthy recipes.

Bill and Agi Lidle travel throughout the country sharing their message of "Living A Healthy Lifestyle Together."

If you are interested in attending a "Fresh Start" class, would like to know where Bill and Agi are speaking, receive a copy of the Healing VOICE newsletter, or speak with Agi personally call:

480-948-3386
or email: ablhealth@aol.com